W9-BKQ-531

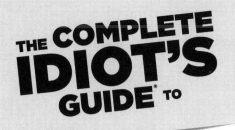

Weight Training

Illustrated

Fourth Edition

by Deidre Johnson, Jonathan Cane, and Joe Glickman

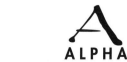

ALPHA

A member of Penguin Group (USA) Inc.

To our families, who gave us the passion to lift and the chutzpah to write.
—Deidre, Jonathan, and Joe

ALPHA BOOKS

Published by Penguin Group (USA) Inc.

Penguin Group (USA) Inc., 375 Hudson Street, New York, New York 10014, USA • Penguin Group (Canada), 90 Eglinton Avenue East, Suite 700, Toronto, Ontario M4P 2Y3, Canada (a division of Pearson Penguin Canada Inc.) • Penguin Books Ltd., 80 Strand, London WC2R 0RL, England • Penguin Ireland, 25 St. Stephen's Green, Dublin 2, Ireland (a division of Penguin Books Ltd.) • Penguin Group (Australia), 250 Camberwell Road, Camberwell, Victoria 3124, Australia (a division of Pearson Australia Group Pty. Ltd.) • Penguin Books India Pvt. Ltd., 11 Community Centre, Panchsheel Park, New Delhi—110 017, India • Penguin Group (NZ), 67 Apollo Drive, Rosedale, North Shore, Auckland 1311, New Zealand (a division of Pearson New Zealand Ltd.) • Penguin Books (South Africa) (Pty.) Ltd., 24 Sturdee Avenue, Rosebank, Johannesburg 2196, South Africa • Penguin Books Ltd., Registered Offices: 80 Strand, London WC2R 0RL, England

International Standard Book Number: 978-1-61564-228-1
Library of Congress Catalog Card Number: 2012941779

14   13   12   8 7 6 5 4 3 2 1

Interpretation of the printing code: The rightmost number of the first series of numbers is the year of the book's printing; the rightmost number of the second series of numbers is the number of the book's printing. For example, a printing code of 12-1 shows that the first printing occurred in 2012.

Printed in the United States of America

Note: This publication contains the opinions and ideas of its authors. It is intended to provide helpful and informative material on the subject matter covered. It is sold with the understanding that the authors and publisher are not engaged in rendering professional services in the book. If the reader requires personal assistance or advice, a competent professional should be consulted.

The authors and publisher specifically disclaim any responsibility for any liability, loss, or risk, personal or otherwise, which is incurred as a consequence, directly or indirectly, of the use and application of any of the contents of this book.

Most Alpha books are available at special quantity discounts for bulk purchases for sales promotions, premiums, fund-raising, or educational use. Special books, or book excerpts, can also be created to fit specific needs.

For details, write: Special Markets, Alpha Books, 375 Hudson Street, New York, NY 10014.

Publisher: *Mike Sanders*

Executive Managing Editor: *Billy Fields*

Senior Acquisitions Editor: *Tom Stevens*

Development Editor: *Michael Thomas*

Senior Production Editor: *Janette Lynn*

Copy Editor: *Krista Hansing Editorial Services, Inc.*

Cover Designer: *William Thomas*

Book Designers: *William Thomas, Rebecca Batchelor*

Indexer: *Tonya Heard*

Layout: *Brian Massey*

Proofreader: *John Etchison*

ALWAYS LEARNING   PEARSON

Contents

Appendixes

Introduction

We've all seen the infomercials on TV in which some model using the Superduper Tummy Tuck machine has achieved his statuesque body by supposedly using this gizmo for 20 minutes every other day. Never mind that the body-beautiful model is an out-of-work actor who has spent three hours a day working out for the last 10 years. The selling point behind virtually all these "quick-and-easy" fitness devices is that honing your body into a figure Michelangelo would be eager to sculpt is basically effortless. This, of course, isn't the case.

Getting into peak physical shape takes time and effort. That's the bad news. The good news is that you have plenty of time to realize the strong and supple physique you've always wanted. Why? Getting into and then staying in shape is a lifelong process, not something you do in frenetic preparation for your twentieth high school reunion or to look good at the beach. Done properly, strength training is an important step in a process of learning how to restore your body's natural gifts—gifts that are often stymied by our busy modern lives.

While we can't guarantee that reading this book will turn you into a magazine cover model, we feel quite confident that if you follow our advice and implement it correctly, you will look and feel better than you've ever felt before—it just might take longer than 20 minutes.

How This Book Is Organized

This book is a complete guide to strength training, but it is also a primer on getting and staying in shape on a more comprehensive basis. We concentrate on lifting weights, but we hope to impress upon you the importance of proper nutrition, posture, stretching, and cardiovascular exercise as well. Strength training will get you strong; implementing these other aspects will get you fit. We present you with everything the beginner needs to know to make the introduction to weightlifting as painless (literally and figuratively) as possible. You learn about everything from shopping for a gym to setting up your first exercise program to pushing through plateaus as you progress.

We've divided the book into two major parts:

In **Part 1, Gearing Up,** we fill you in on everything you need to know before you begin a weightlifting program, including some important advice about how you really can't afford *not* to work out. Chapter 1 tells you all you need to know about choosing the right gym, and we also give you the lowdown on how to equip your home gym, if that's the route you take. We help you choose the right duds for your workout, too. In Chapter 2, we move on to the basics of a proper diet. Chapter 3 addresses the dreaded but often necessary visit to the doctor, as well as safety issues in the gym. In Chapter 4, we move into the gym and begin stretching.

It's funny how many people who start lifting have little or no idea what muscles they're working. "I want to work these things," they say, pointing to their deltoids. That's where **Part 2, The Workout,** comes in. Chapter 5 gives you a rundown on what to expect when you begin lifting. We underscore the importance of proper form and technique—the foundation of any program. Chapters 6 through 12 are the guts of the how-to section, with each chapter addressing a specific muscle group. Exercises are accompanied by photos and a thorough explanation of what to do. When you've learned the nuances of the equipment, the exercises, and the philosophy behind working out, you can use the guidelines in Chapter 13 to determine which exercises to include in your routine, based on your goals and time constraints. You'll also learn what to do if things aren't working out the way you expected. Chapter 14 clues you in on some of the most popular and effective trends in strength training. Finally, in Chapter 15, we discuss strategies for staying in shape even if you can't make it to the gym.

Extras

To make the learning experience as easy and as fun as possible, we've highlighted lots of tips and facts along the way. Look for the following elements throughout the book to guide you:

FLEX FACTS

These sidebars include interesting tidbits and anecdotes. They're not essential for you to have a safe or effective workout, but you should find them informative and sometimes amusing.

DEFINITION

These sidebars provide you with definitions of new terms introduced in the text. By adding them to your gymspeak vocabulary, you might not lift any better, but you will be better informed.

SPOT ME

These sidebars provide tips and pointers to help make your lifting more effective. Think of them as having a personal trainer giving you help throughout your workout. They highlight little things that you might not otherwise notice.

WEIGHT A MINUTE

These sidebars highlight safety issues important to your health and welfare. The gym can be a dangerous and intimidating place if you don't know what to expect. Read these cautions carefully to ensure that your workout is pain free.

Acknowledgments

Writing a book is a little like building a beautiful body: it's a great idea with many rich rewards, but it boils down to plain old hard work. The three of us—friends when we started, better friends when we finished—enjoyed working on this project, but plenty of times we would rather have been doing something else. Of course, writing this book would have been far more difficult without the invaluable input of quite a few people.

Thanks to Body Reserve, in Brooklyn, New York, for the use of the facility for the photo shoot. We're grateful to Gene Schaffer of ARC Athletics for his expertise with kettlebells and medicine balls, as well as the invaluable help of Maria Simone.

Also, our models are more than just buffed bods and pretty faces—they're all fine athletes and better friends. Special thanks to Susan Stanley, Laura Galbraith, Elizabeth Ann Corkum, Nicole Sin Quee, Gary Berard, Terence Gerchberg, and Conrad Kiffin.

Special thanks from Deidre to her father and sister for their endless faith in her and to Laura Giovanella for her patience and support.

Jonathan would like to thank a few of his teachers—Bob Otto, John Wygand, Bob Perez, and Ralph Carpinelli—without whom this book would contain far fewer big words and sophisticated ideas. Thanks to his training mates for making him work; the athletes he coaches for keeping him honest; his co-authors for tolerating him; and, most of all, his wife, Nicole, for her support and patience, and his son, Simon, for being adorable and the same weight as a kettlebell.

Last, but not least, Joe wishes to thank his lovely, literate wife, Beth, and darling 15-year-old daughter, Willa. Most of all, he'd like to thank his co-authors, Jonathan, a terrible mountain biker but great coach, and "D," a beautiful woman who gets downright ugly when she wins World Powerlifting Championships. Without their wit and wisdom, he would still be wandering lost in the fitness forest.

Trademarks

Gearing Up

In this first part, we fill you in on everything you need to know before you begin a weightlifting program, including some important advice about how you really can't afford *not* to work out. Many people want to work out but feel intimidated by the newness of this foreign place called a gym, full of sweaty strangers and loud music. In fact, a gym is a social place where you're likely to make good friends. In the following four chapters, we familiarize you with the nuances of the gym so those first days are largely anxiety free.

Look Before You Lift

In This Chapter

- Finding the gym for you
- Getting help: the lowdown on personal trainers
- Choosing home exercise equipment wisely
- Learning the ABCs of free weights
- Dressing for success in the gym

In one episode of Seinfeld, an obnoxious, no-talent (and not very muscular) comedian tells the slender Jerry Seinfeld that he's gotten so big from lifting weights that his suits no longer fit him. "I'm huge!" he brags. "You really oughta lift." Jerry replies, "Why?" This basic bit of logic throws the "pumped" lifter for a loop. "Don't know," he says quizzically.

Well, there are more good reasons to lift weights than there are good sitcoms on television. But before you leap into your workouts, it's important to take a look around the gym. In this chapter, we help you decide between working out at home and joining a gym, and we give you tips on shopping for either. Plus, we help you choose clothes that maximize both form and function. Read on!

Eenie, Meenie, Miney, Mo

This obvious bit of advice takes many people by surprise: the more specific your fitness goals, the easier it is to pick a gym that suits your needs. In other words, are you there to pump iron, or are you interested in taking group classes or yoga? Are you looking for swimming, boxing, or basketball opportunities? Is taking a sauna a big plus or no big deal? Remember, if your gym has these amenities and you choose not to use them, you're likely subsidizing someone else's use of them.

As long as we're talking about the obvious, be sure that the gym you join has hours that work for you. We know one gym in Brooklyn that sits over a synagogue and must close on the Sabbath and Jewish holidays.

"Gosh," you may be saying, "I just want to find a gym and get in shape, not choose a four-year college." Don't worry. In the pages that follow, we help you identify what to look for in an institution of higher fitness, factoring in everything from your legal rights to your creature comforts.

Neatness—or, at Least, Cleanliness—Counts!

Surveying a gym is a bit like looking for a home. But instead of looking for closet space and listening for street noise, you want to focus on the general cleanliness of the gym area and locker rooms, as well as the quality of the equipment. When you enter a new gym for inspection, don your white gloves and prepare to judge!

Look for the following in the gym area:

- Take a good look at the general condition of the equipment. For example, are the cables on the gym equipment in good repair, or are they frayed?

- Check out the equipment's manufacturer. If it's Life Fitness, Cybex, Precor, or Nautilus, that's a good sign. Stu's, Herb's, or Skippy's should send up a warning signal.

- Is the upholstery covering the equipment worn or torn? If the equipment looks like the inside of a honky-tonk, consider other alternatives.

- Check out the dumbbells—the handheld weights you'll soon become familiar with. Are they the plated variety, which hold up well, or the hexagonal type, which tend to bend and rust?

Now go into the locker room and evaluate the following:

- Is the room clean?

- Are the lockers large enough to accommodate your gear? We've been to gyms where fitting your clothes into a skinny locker is like squeezing a thick English muffin into a narrow-slotted toaster. In winter, when you'll be toting even more clothes, this toaster phenomenon gets worse. So buyer beware.

- Are lockers available for rent? Renting a locker allows you to leave stuff at the gym, like a weight belt, shampoo, deodorant, or a hair dryer—a clutch item if you'll be heading for the office or the movies after your workout.

- Are the stalls in the bathroom clean? Or is the place like the restroom at an interstate rest stop? Do the stalls have toilet paper?

- Ditto for the shower stalls. A nice, hot, relaxing shower after a workout is supremely satisfying, unless the space is a moldy mess reserved for jungle explorers and cattle rustlers. Also, it's not a bad idea to check the water pressure. A dribbling showerhead just doesn't get it done.

- What about the upkeep of the steam room, sauna, and whirlpool? Again, these are excellent features—provided that they're fit for human enjoyment.

Do You Have X, Y, and Z?

Gyms are a bit like restaurants: the basic product is the same, but the pomp and circumstance vary widely. To some, the only factors of concern when selecting a gym are whether they have enough equipment and whether the price is right. Everything else is window dressing.

Consider a "musclehead" gym we know in Brooklyn that's so austere and grungy it's almost cool. Inside, large, animated men with biceps the size of cantaloupes hoist free weights like NFL linemen tossing back spare ribs. The grunting and groaning is so intense that you'd almost think you were listening to natural childbirth. Shampoo and conditioner in the shower stalls? Get real! Patrons are lucky there's water in the water fountain. Nevertheless, the gym has 9 million pounds of free weights, and the annual membership is about the cost of dinner for nine at McDonald's. For some, that's just what the doctor ordered.

On the other hand, if you prefer a more pristine setting, or if the sight of a spider in the bathroom sends you scurrying for a vaccination, you may want to consider a classier establishment.

Let's look at the amenities you may want to consider, realizing ahead of time that the more you get, the more you'll pay!

Ambience

Although you rarely hear the word *ambience* used to describe a gym, each establishment has its own feel, character, and mood. How do you feel when you enter a club? Are you comfortable there, or do you feel like racing out like a prisoner pardoned from jail? It's good practice to trust your initial impression, because often your gut-level feeling determines whether you stick with the place.

After working out in her neighborhood gym for many years, Deidre decided to join a gym that was closer to her job. Deidre appreciates the finer things in life but cares little whether her gym has soft hankies in the ladies' room. However, the new club she joined had old, run-down equipment and a decrepit locker room, and played awful music really loud. Even for a tough gym rat like her, the squalid scene detracted from the quality of her workouts. Before too long, she was back in her bare-bones gym, which suddenly seemed much more appealing.

Know this: very few gyms let you tour their facility on your own. Usually, you'll be chaperoned by a salesperson whose job it is to get you to join. Keep this in mind, and don't let anyone rush you through a suspect area of the gym. In addition, don't let anyone hurry you into signing a contract on the spot if you're on the fence about whether to join. The salesperson might tell you the club is running a "special" sale, but more often than not, this select opportunity happens as frequently as a full moon—like every month! In other words, if you're not ready to buy, we assure you that another promotional deal will come along sooner rather than later.

Curiously (or not), the same gym has a different feel depending on when you visit. Why? Gym regulars cycle through in predictable shifts: there's the prework crowd, the midmorning- and afternoon-lull set, the post-work rush, and the late-night revelers. That's why it's best to check out the gym you're examining at the hour you'll be working out. There's no sense in looking at a mellow, half-empty gym at noon if you're going to be rubbing elbows during peak evening hours with dozens of other patrons jockeying for the equipment.

If the place is too trendy or too low rent, or too loud or eerily silent for your tastes, or if the price is right but the neighborhood is wrong, remember that you've got options. Be sure you check out one of the other 14,000-plus gyms out there. You're no doubt bound to find one that feels right for you.

SPOT ME

For you web surfers, a great resource when shopping for a gym is www.healthclubs.com. Narrow your search by entering your zip code and the type of facility you're looking for, and the site will instantly supply you with a list of gyms that fit your needs.

Bond or Bust

Here's a situation you may not have considered: on Monday you go to the gym to work your chest and back; on Wednesday you're back to do arms and shoulders when you learn that the gym is going belly up. Out of business. Chapter 11. Gone. Good-bye.

If the gym you join is bonded, you're guaranteed at least a partial refund. A bond is a contract between the state and the gym that ensures a gym member will have some financial recourse if the facility goes out of business before his or her membership expires. Roughly half the states in the country require that a fitness center carry a bond of at least $50,000. If a bond is required in your state, the gym must have proof that it has one if you ask. Again, if a bonded gym bites the dust, this doesn't mean you'll get a full refund, but it's insurance that you'll get at least some money back. If your gym is not bonded, there's not much you can do.

You might think that calling your state's chamber of commerce or Better Business Bureau to see if your gym has a bond might seem like overkill, but gyms go out of business all the time, sometimes under shady circumstances. Deidre once worked as a massage therapist at a health club that one day closed its doors as suddenly as a three-card monty dealer folds his cardboard table. Even worse, in the days preceding this unannounced event, the owners offered tremendous deals on multiyear memberships. Obviously, these guys were trying to rake in as much cash as possible before closing up shop. (The only recourse any member had was to break in and hock the furniture. Try selling a used leg extension machine on the street—it's not a pretty sight.)

Your Escape Clause

You've got another good reason to read your gym contract carefully before you sign. Most states provide some sort of "buyer's remorse" clause in the contract that gives you anywhere from 24 to 72 hours to cancel your membership without being penalized. Similarly, a clause in the contract may cover you if you move out of the area or are injured before your contract runs out. Some gyms allow members to "freeze" their memberships for certain periods—after having a baby, after being injured, to take a long vacation, and so on. And often if you move a significant distance from your gym (usually 25 miles), you'll be entitled to a prorated refund.

We realize that you didn't buy this book to read about contracts, but know this: you can often have riders added to your contract. Remember that smiling salespeople often have more flexibility in what they can offer than they let on. You might be able to negotiate a family membership deal or a group discount if you recruit new members. If the gym doesn't offer discounts, you may be able to add another month to your membership or have a personal training session tossed into the mix. Remember, if you don't ask, you'll never know what accommodations you may be able to obtain.

For example, if you regularly travel out of town for weeks or months at a time, you can probably have the contract amended to account for this. Alternatively, your club might be affiliated with a national chain or organization (IHRSA, the International Health, Racquet and Sportsclub Association, is the largest and most reputable) that allows you to work out at another gym while you're on the road—usually free or at a discounted rate.

Just How Much Is This Going to Cost?

Pick a number between $99 and $9,999, and you've narrowed the price of joining a gym. In other words, the cost of a health club membership can vary widely, even within the same gym, because there are peak and off-peak memberships, month-to-month or annual contracts, and several options in between.

What's this about a month-to-month contract, you ask? Well, most clubs offer them, and they have several advantages over an annual contract:

- You don't have to lay out a lot of cash when you join.
- If you're not comfortable with the gym, just finish out the month, and you won't feel a financial pinch.
- Ditto if you move, travel a lot, get injured, or are abducted by aliens.

But there's always another side of the coin, isn't there? Here are some of the disadvantages of having a month-to-month contract:

- If you continue to work out, it will end up costing you more at the end of the year.
- An "initiation fee" usually is associated with month-to-month memberships but is often waived or nonexistent with annuals.

Give Me Exercise or Give Me Death

Okay, we said we were done talking about your gym contract, but we think you should know a few more things. Here's an incident that illustrates a bogus practice employed by a gym in Brooklyn. This particular club allows you to pay on a monthly basis by automatically deducting the fee from your checking account. However, when a patron we know wanted to quit, she had to mail a certified letter. Then the gym could charge her another monthly fee until 30 days after it received the letter. In short, they made getting out of the contract as easy as settling a debt with the Mafia. Protect yourself by understanding the club's policy on cancellations. Many require 30 to 60 days' written notice.

As a consumer, you have rights when you purchase a membership from a health club. (Remember that the contract not only spells out your commitment to the gym, but also protects you against fraudulent acts by the owners.) In fact, most states have specific statutes that spell out consumers' rights when it comes to health clubs.

That said, we don't mean to imply that most gyms are out to rook you. Far from it. Most gyms are legitimate businesses that make a profit by providing good service. But as in all things, when it comes to signing on the dotted line and handing over a check—buyer beware!

Evaluating the Trainers

Trainers present yet another of those good news/bad news deals. Well-trained, knowledgeable, concerned fitness experts are an invaluable asset in the gym. They can help motivate you, offer advice on everything from nutrition to stretching, and guide you through your workout. If you've got the will—and sometimes even if you don't—a good trainer has the way. The bad news, however, is that the staff members at many fitness centers aren't always well trained, informed, or concerned.

Depending on a trainer's qualifications, reputation, and demand, expect to pay anywhere from $25 to $150 an hour for a training session. (Introductory sessions are often available to new members.) Some trainers trim the price if you work with a partner.

Keep in mind that anyone who walks and talks can call him- or herself a "personal trainer," "exercise physiologist," or "fitness instructor." Scary as it sounds, in most states, you need a license to cut hair but not to be a personal trainer.

The better establishments are staffed with trainers who have college degrees in exercise physiology, biomechanics, or other health sciences. In others, the instructors may have no laurels to rest on other than their beefy pectoral muscles. In-house certifications offered by some of the big national chains are as tough to pass as Basket Weaving 101. Essentially, their requirements are minimal, and the certification is just a way to let the gym tell folks that its staff is certified.

WEIGHT A MINUTE

Don't be impressed just because a trainer is "certified." Clubs often have their own certifications—usually just a gimmick to pump up the appearance of their staff's credentials. Look for nationally recognized certifications or college degrees.

It's a good idea to check with the salespeople about the staff's qualifications. Scores of alphabet-soup certifications exist. The most respected is the American College of Sports Medicine (ACSM), although other organizations, such as the National Strength and Conditioning Association (NSCA), the National Academy of Sports Medicine (NASM), and the American Council on Exercise (ACE) also have certification programs.

If you do opt to work with a trainer—even for a few sessions, to help you get started—be sure your trainer is not only qualified, but insured as well. We sincerely hope it never happens, but if you are injured due to a trainer's neglect, you'll want your trainer to have liability insurance.

Now that you've had a chance to evaluate the idea of making a gym a part of your life, let's take a look at another viable option: creating a home gym that works for you.

There's No Place Like Home

Okay, let's say you're starting to think that working out at home is the way to go for you. What now? Well, now you've got to look into the future a bit and anticipate some of the challenges you may face. Don't worry, we'll walk you through it!

One important disadvantage of working out at home is that you have no spotter, a kind soul who will be sure you don't drop a weight on your head. Most home gym equipment is designed to minimize (or eliminate) this problem, but the potential still exists. Let's take a look.

Recognizing and Avoiding Home Gym Pitfalls

It sounds perfect, doesn't it? If you have gym equipment at home, you can work out in privacy on your own schedule. No driving to the gym, no waiting for equipment, no need to worry about closing time. What could be better?

Before you assume that home is where the exercise is, consider a few built-in pitfalls. Perhaps the most important one concerns safety—an issue we return to throughout this book. If you're working out at home, you're almost always also working out alone, and that can be dangerous.

For instance, one day many moons ago, Joe came home and found his father stuck upside down like a bat hanging helplessly in a pair of inversion boots (an odd but once-popular piece of home gym equipment). One can only imagine what this poor old man would have done had no one come along to extricate him from his perilous predicament. Another time, Mr. Glickman was benching a modest amount of weight and was unable to press the bar from his chest. Stuck like a mouse in a trap, he slowly, painfully, rolled the weight toward his knees until he was able to squeeze out from under it. Although these examples are humorous, each year several deaths from weight training occur. Usually the cause of death is suffocation from dropping the bar across the neck during the bench press. These kinds of stories are virtually nonexistent in a gym, where patrons and trainers typically rush to your assistance.

Needless to say, because you are alone, you need to take extra care to read the instructions that come with your home unit. If you don't understand something, don't hesitate to call the manufacturer. Many units come with a video, too. Take the time to watch it—it could spare you an injury.

What You Need and What It Costs

Assuming that you're like us and plan on working out until you're put out to pasture, setting up a home gym is more economical over the long term. (Actually, working out in a pasture is rather appealing as well!) Of course, if your shiny, high-tech piece of equipment becomes the featured item in a garage sale, you've been penny-wise and weight-foolish. Let's examine the cost of a complete home gym. We start with the equipment, which should include these three components:

- *Cardiovascular* **equipment.** You need some type of machine—stationary bike, rowing machine, or treadmill—that gets your ticker ticking.

- **Resistance equipment.** This apparatus helps you build muscle.

- **An exercise mat.** We discuss stretching at length in Chapter 4, but for now, know that working on your flexibility should be an integral part of any fitness regimen. A mat makes stretching and abdominal exercises far more comfortable.

DEFINITION

Cardiovascular exercise is any activity that elevates your heart rate over a sustained period of time. Your body's cardiovascular system includes your heart and lungs.

Cardio Action

What type of cardio machine should you buy? And how much can you expect to spend? Let's do a little imaginary shopping.

A stationary bike with bells and whistles like the LifeCycle can cost as much as $2,000, or you can spend as little as $300 for a basic stationary model. Here's the catch-22: if you're not sure you'll use it, it's best to start with the cheaper model. However, if you're planning to become the next Lance Armstrong, the sturdier machine is preferable. Years ago, one of Jonathan's future teammates on his cycling team, a guy who hadn't cycled or exercised in years, started riding on a low-rent stationary bike he bought for a song. Before long, he had ridden it so often that he'd ground it into pencil shavings. Afterward, he started riding on the road and went on to become one of the best riders in the state. If you already have a bicycle, a fine way to work out indoors is to buy a contraption that allows you to remove the front wheel and ride your bike indoors as a stationary model. State-of-the art models can go for as much as $1,500, but such an apparatus usually goes for between $100 and $250.

If biking isn't your thing, let your feet do the walking and buy a treadmill. As is true for the stationary bike, you have a whole range of options for a treadmill, ranging in price from $500 to $5,000. Again, if you're going to use it regularly, it's far better to drop four figures on a solid machine. Three brands we particularly like are TRUE, Life Fitness, and Precor.

Don't like to run or bike? A variety of other machines help get your heart pumping, including the Concept II rowing machine, NordicTrack cross-country ski simulators, stair climbers like the StairMaster, and the increasingly popular elliptical trainers that provide a great low-impact workout.

The Weight Stuff

Now that we've explored the world of cardio equipment, it's time to discuss the meat and potatoes (or, better yet, the broiled fish and brown rice—but we'll get to the diet stuff later in the book) of the home gym: resistance equipment.

Here's what to look for in an "all-in-one" unit:

- **A variety of exercises.** No matter how effective the exercise, a continuing routine of the same few exercises will leave you feeling bored.

- **Ease of movement from one exercise to another.** If transitioning from one exercise to another is difficult or time-consuming, you're not likely to use the machine. Or if you do use it, you're not likely to get a good workout.

- **Enough resistance to grow with you as you get stronger.** Right now the lightest weight on the machine may be just a little too heavy for you to lift, but—as hard as it may be to imagine now—you won't be in that position for long. You'll get stronger, and you'll want a machine that will help you do just that. If you have to do 38 repetitions of an exercise to tax yourself, you need to increase the weight.

- **An objective measure of your progress.** You need a way to tell how strong you're getting from one week to the next. Progress is inspirational. If you see that you're able to do 10 more repetitions of a particular exercise, you're more likely to keep at it.

Quite a few multifunction strength-training machines on the market are versatile, sturdy, and safe. Of course, each has its advantages and disadvantages.

The Power of Free Weights

If you want to go "old school," you can buy an adjustable bench ($300 to $500) and a set of free weights, and knock yourself out (but not literally!). Although initially this might seem like the simpler, less expensive way to go, the costs quickly add up, and it can become far more expensive than you might have anticipated. Furthermore, for the novice, using free weights in an unsupervised setting makes us more than a wee bit nervous. Still, a free weight setup at home can work quite well if you take the time to learn the rules and then follow them.

Now for the cost. You probably don't want or need a full set of dumbbells in your home. A good option is a pair of adjustable dumbbells such as the PowerBlock. Selling for roughly $200, the PowerBlock enables you to easily and quickly adjust the weight of the barbell from 5 to 45 pounds. Newcomers in the adjustable dumbbell field include Probell and Versabell, each of which offers similar features.

When shopping for a bar and weights (also known as plates), you have a few options. "Olympic" bars, found in just about every gym, are 7 feet long and weigh 45 pounds. (Shorter, lighter bars are also available.)

Plates are available in increments of 2.5 through 100 pounds. Figure on spending about 25¢ per pound—a sum that adds up if you're a budding moose. Throw on a pair of collars (the clips that secure the plates at either end of the bar), and you're good to go for just about any of the exercises we describe in future chapters. We say "just about" because a few are unsafe to do without a spotter. We note the risky ones so you don't end up with an imprint of a barbell on your nose.

As we've said, unless you're willing to spend a small fortune, you'll never duplicate the wide range of equipment a good gym can offer (to say nothing of the guidance trainers can provide). However, even the best gym in the solar system does you no good if you don't use it. Working out in a gym is the most reliable way to build a fitter body, but a home gym is certainly the next best thing.

Strain in Style

What you wear to the gym is an issue of the utmost importance that really doesn't matter. By that, we mean that if it's comfortable, allows a full range of motion, and adheres to gym regulations, you could wear a tuxedo with tails or an evening gown and be good to go. This sounds ridiculous—and it is—but a few years ago, a swift runner ran the New York City Marathon in a tuxedo jacket and shorts. (He discarded the black shoes and went with a pair of Nikes.)

So while you could work out effectively in a burlap bag, what you wear is of enormous personal relevance to who you are and what kind of statement you want to make—if you want to make any at all. Are you flashy or modest? A Lycra proponent or a fan of organic cotton? Do you go with the neon lime green bike jersey and large silver hoop earrings, or stick with the ripped T-shirt you wore when you went fishing with your Uncle Sylvester? In this section, we outline your options and make some recommendations about the right workout clothes for you.

Do Clothes Make the Athlete?

Although we adhere to the philosophy of "to each his own," some people's workout attire can be perplexing. Deidre and Joe frequently find themselves working out next to a hulking guy who can lift a compact car and the kitchen sink. However, no matter how hot it gets, he wears an XXL sweatshirt and long, baggy pants. Although he has the body of an NFL linebacker, the self-effacing chap refuses to show skin. Another full-bodied woman they know wears skintight outfits that would make Beyoncé blush.

Even more confusing is the dignified gent who works out in the same immaculate outfit every time: red tank top, blue shorts, white socks, and white sneakers. This is a perfectly fine outfit, but we're dying to know whether he has two dozen of the same items (and if so, why?) or whether he's just laundering the same combination after every workout? These, dear reader, are some of the questions that can weigh on a petty man's mind.

Simply put, picking an outfit to exercise in at the gym can be purely perfunctory or a fair bit of fun. We have more than a few biases on the subject that we'll gladly share with you in the following pages, but the bottom line is this: if the garment fits, wear it.

The Threads

The best workout clothing consists of any combination of comfortable garments that allow freedom of movement and a modicum of modesty. When Joe began competing in kayak marathons with international paddlers, he was initially surprised to see that the majority of the world-class Australian and South African kayakers he raced against wore baggy T-shirts—quite a contrast to the Americans, who often wore tight tank tops. Why the baggy look? These guys had chiseled upper bodies straight from central casting. The answer: it's comfortable, mate! In other words, if you've got the goods, why compromise comfort for vanity? Before you could say *rip curl*, many of the Americans started wearing extra-large as well.

Here's a basic list of acceptable gym threads:

- Sweatpants
- Shorts
- Leggings/tights
- T-shirts

- Tank tops
- Sports bras
- Sweatshirts

Although some people find wearing a tank top too revealing, keep in mind that it's always a good idea to concentrate on the muscle groups you're working, so if you're concentrating on your upper body, a tank top may be just the thing. Not only is it easier to focus on the task at hand if you can see the muscle actually lengthening and contracting, but it can also be a good motivational tool to see your muscles grow before your eyes—a phenomenon known as the *pump*.

DEFINITION

Lifters often refer to the swelling in a muscle immediately after lifting as the **pump**. Although it appears that the muscle is growing as you lift, what you see is actually the muscle becoming temporarily engorged with blood—not the same thing as when the muscles themselves grow.

When working her upper body, Deidre usually wears a sports bra and sweatpants, and she dons a T-shirt and shorts when she works her lower body.

Joe, who has arguably the largest collection of race T-shirts in North America, tends to modify his attire according to the aerobic activity he's doing that day. If he's going to run and lift, he wears jogging shorts and brings an extra T-shirt (no problem there). If he's going to cycle or use the Concept II rower, he's likely to wear bike shorts and, you guessed it, a T-shirt. Also, on "leg" day, he prefers bike shorts because they offer better support when he does squats.

Jonathan, the triathlon coach who has been known to dine in trendy Manhattan restaurants in a black warm-up suit (arguing that, strictly speaking, it is a suit), doesn't really care what he's wearing as long as he's working out. In fact, Jonathan probably would lift in a lobster bib if he forgot to pack one of his 900 T-shirts.

Women's Wear

Today most women who exercise regularly wear a sports bra and T-shirt with sweats or shorts. The three points to remember about sports bras are proper fit, comfort, and structure.

- **Fit.** When selecting a sports bra, always try it on before you get to the gym. When you've got it on, clap your hands overhead; if the plastic band moves up your chest, it's too tight. You don't want to start working out and discover that you're wearing an iron corset that doesn't allow you to breathe. And you don't want to fret about peek-a-boo bosom while you're lying in the middle of a bench or performing another cleavage-revealing exercise.

- **Comfort.** To continue on our sartorial theme, looking good doesn't equal feeling good. Besides, the better you feel when you work out, the more apt you are to keep training!

- **Structure.** Basically, you have two choices in sports bras: compression and encapsulation. Neither sounds terribly forgiving, but the latter tends to be the most comfortable. True to its name, the compression bra presses (read: squishes) the breasts against the chest in a single mass. This style is more appropriate for small- to medium-breasted women. Like a brassiere, the encapsulation type is built to hold each breast in a cup. This works better for full-figured women.

The Treads

If you haven't already noticed, a trip to a well-equipped sporting goods store reveals just how specialized workout gear has become. This is especially true in the footwear realm. In fact, never-throw-out-a-pair-of-running-shoes jocks like Jonathan and Joe each have at least 44 pairs (okay, maybe more, but we don't have time to tally them all). Think we're exaggerating? Here's a basic outline of the footwear you could find in our collective closets:

- Running shoes for the road (lots of them!)

- Trail running shoes

- Cycling shoes for biking on the road

- Cycling shoes for mountain biking and touring

- Basketball shoes

- Tennis shoes

- Cross-training shoes (hybrid sneakers designed to do a bit of everything)

- Water shoes (slipperlike footwear designed for kayakers)

- Approach shoes designed for easy hiking

- Sports sandals

SPOT ME

When buying a new pair of shoes, it's a good idea to try them on in the evening because your feet tend to swell toward the end of the day. What feels good at 9 a.m. might be a wee bit snug at dinnertime.

With the obvious exception of cycling shoes that feature protruding cleats that leave you walking like a petrified tree, most of the previously mentioned footwear is fine for just lifting weights. Remember that many Olympic-level marathon runners have run like the wind barefoot. So although the sport specificity in footwear does have its place, you can wear just about anything as long as it fits and gives you adequate support.

Herein lies the rub. Ideally, your footwear should provide you with ample arch support as well as proper medial (inside aspect of the foot) and lateral (outside) support. If you've ever had any foot pain, your best bet is to go to a store known for its sneaker savvy. Be specific with the salesperson when talking about what you'll be doing in these sneakers. If you know that you're flat-footed (have no arch), *overpronate* (have an exaggerated roll to the inner portion of your foot), or *supinate* (walk on the outer portion), inform the salesperson; sales reps who know what they're doing will recommend shoes designed for those specific conditions. If you don't understand pronation, buy whatever feels best and, over time, monitor where the majority of the wear and tear on your footwear occurs. (If you're a runner, this will quickly become obvious.) Generally, when you're shopping for shoes for weightlifting, a cross-training shoe is your best bet for appropriate support.

DEFINITION

To **overpronate,** as it relates to walking, is to bear most of your weight on the inner portion of your foot. You can often tell by looking at the wear pattern on the soles of your shoes whether you pronate or **supinate,** which means to bear weight on the outer portion of your foot as you walk.

Wrap It Up

One of the neat things about strength training is that you can do it in a sophisticated gym with high-tech equipment or in a bare-bones basement with a bench, a few handheld weights, and plenty of desire. In either setting, however, you bring only what you're wearing and possibly an assortment of goodies that may (or may not) help you get stronger.

We're talking about *weight belts*, wrist and knee wraps, and gloves. Is this stuff necessary? Not really. Can the mere sight of this equipment get you psyched to go to the gym? Possibly. Let's talk a bit about each one, and you can decide for yourself.

Buckle Up!

To belt or not to belt, that's a question that has generated a fair bit of debate among fitness devotees. The good news is that wearing a weight belt reminds you to maintain erect posture while you lift. The bad news is twofold: the belt offers support to the muscles in your lower back and abdomen that you're trying to strengthen, and wearing one can give you a false sense of security that may have you trying to lift more weight than is safe or necessary. Of course, if you have a weak lower back, a belt may be necessary to work out pain free until we can help you strengthen your abdominal and lower back muscles.

DEFINITION

A **weight belt** is made from thick, dense leather and is roughly 6 inches wide. It's buckled securely around your waist just above your hips.

In many ways, wearing a belt offers more psychological comfort than actual aid. If you suffer from low-level chronic back pain, wearing one can be comforting—it's like a heating pad without the heat, if you will. Furthermore, it's like an athlete who rubs the head of the trusty old trainer before taking the field. As they approach an imposing bar loaded with weight, many lifters cinch the buckle one notch tighter, a gesture that gets them psyched for the challenge more than anything else.

During her powerlifting days, Deidre wore a belt. But remember, her sport was about demonstrating strength; your goal in the gym is to gain strength. In other words, her goal was to lift the heaviest weight she possibly could, so wearing a belt while she squatted or deadlifted helped to up her totals. Again, we're concerned about what your *muscles* can do, not what your *gear* can do. Unless you feel that you need to wear a belt, we recommend you don't.

For a belt to offer any significant support, it has to be pulled so tight that you'd barely be able to whistle. By comparison, the corsets worn by female French nobility were as comfy as housedresses. In fact, before Deidre would approach a *squat* or deadlift, it would take two strong people to yank on her belt to get it tight enough to give her sufficient support. Hauling a marlin into a fishing boat wasn't as much of a struggle.

DEFINITION

The **squat** is a great full-body exercise that involves performing a deep knee bend with a barbell across your back. Sounds intimidating, but fret not; we take you through the proper execution of this movement in Chapter 7.

It's a Wrap

You can use two kinds of wraps in the gym: wrist wraps and knee wraps. Wrist wraps are shorter and affixed with Velcro. The longer knee wraps are cinched by tucking the wrap under itself and pulling.

Remember, for wraps to be effective, they have to be pulled pretty tight. There are only a few good reasons to wear wrist wraps:

- If you've recently suffered a wrist injury, you may need the support.

- If you have a tendency to *hyperextend* your wrists while you perform a bench press, it's a good idea to wrap. Otherwise, you could drop the bar.

DEFINITION

To **hyperextend** means to bend a body part beyond its normal anatomical or neutral position. For example, if you straighten your arm to lock your elbow, it will end up in a straight line. People who are called "double-jointed" can lock their elbow beyond that straight-line position so that it looks as though their elbow is bending in the opposite direction. This is called hyperextension of your elbow.

Knee wraps? We're generally against them. These mummifying wraps are usually worn to support you when you're performing squats or using the leg press or leg extension machine. (For descriptions of these exercises, see Chapter 7.) We don't like knee wraps, for the same reason we're generally against weight belts. Unless you're squatting or pressing a ton of weight, a person with healthy knees who wears them is wasting his or her time—or worse.

The reason you do these exercises in the first place is to strengthen the muscles around the knee joint. When you wrap your knees, you remove a significant amount of the workload from the muscles and transfer it to the wraps. Simply put, wearing knee wraps defeats the purpose of the exercise.

Here's where people get confused. Wearing wraps helps you lift more weight, which should be good, right? Wrong! Being able to lift more weight is good only if it comes as the result of your muscles getting stronger, not because you've fortified yourself with wraps.

This "might makes right" logic highlights an important point: your lifting should be about *getting* strong, not *seeming* strong. This move-as-much-weight-as-possible syndrome, which afflicts men far more than it does women, is counterproductive to health and is as misguided as erecting an ornate roof before you've built a sound foundation.

We can hear the dissenters saying, "If I lift more with the wraps, my leg muscles won't get injured and I'll get stronger faster." Nice try. Just because your securely wrapped knees can handle an increased load doesn't mean your back or other body parts can. Ironically, wrapping your knees to protect this complex and vulnerable joint may actually end up jeopardizing your safety rather than ensuring it.

Finger Wraps

A noncontroversial option in the lifting game is wearing gloves. Weightlifting gloves, which typically cost around $10, have padded palms and cut-off fingers for ventilation and dexterity. Gloves are good if you look at calluses with disdain, and they can come in handy during certain abusive exercises such as chin-ups and lat pull-downs, which you'll read more about in later chapters.

When Deidre started lifting 20-something years ago, she used gloves until she realized that her feel for the weight improved without them. What does "feel for the weight" mean? Many experienced lifters feel that the more contact they have with the bar, the easier it is to lift the weight. Try both and see for yourself.

Like Deidre, Jonathan and Joe go gloveless. A kayaker whose hands are usually callused and cracked from gripping a paddle hours a day in saltwater, Joe finds that the calluses he's built from lifting help fortify his mitts while paddling.

If you decide to don gloves, try to find a pair with a grippy texture on the palms, and be sure they fit your hands snugly without restricting your movement.

Pads

Instead of gloves, some folks prefer pads, which are small, flat, neoprene squares held in the palms like mini-potholders. Not only do they offer the same comfort and improved grip as gloves, but you also don't have to worry about sweaty-palm syndrome. The downside is that, because you have to carry them around, they tend to disappear like socks in a dryer. Jonathan has collected enough pads from his gym's lost and found to tile Madison Square Garden.

Straps

Straps are another common piece of paraphernalia you'll see in the gym. Made of sturdy, nonstretch material, straps are worn around the wrists and then wrapped around the bar you plan to lift. The purpose of straps is to ease the burden on the gripping muscles in your hands and forearms that often fatigue before the larger working muscles.

Take exercises such as deadlifts, pull-ups, and cable rows, which we explain in depth in Chapter 8. These exercises all involve movements that tax large muscles and hence require you to lift a fair bit of weight. Overusing straps can prevent those hand and forearm muscles from becoming stronger, but straps are useful when a weak grip inhibits you from completing the exercise, a common occurrence if you're lifting a lot of weight.

As you may have gathered by now, we're not big proponents of gadgets that make your exercises easier. Still, when you spend enough time at the gym, you'll see tremendously strong people who lift with a weight belt, wrist and knee straps, and gloves. What's up with that?

People who lift a lot often have developed their own habits—good and bad—over many years of experimentation. However, when you start out, it's important to establish good habits, to lift with sound technique and with as little interference as possible—just you, the weight, knowledge, and plenty of desire.

The Least You Need to Know

- A good gym is the sum total of its parts. Know what to look for, and you won't regret your choice.
- Not all trainers are created equal. Learn which degrees are worth more than the paper they're printed on.
- Setting up a home gym may be more cost effective than paying a gym membership—assuming that you use it.
- Your workout gear should look good and feel better.
- When buying shoes, let fit and function be your guide.
- Weight belts, wrist and knee wraps, and gloves can help or hinder you. Use them with care.

Food for Thought

In This Chapter

- Eating: what and when
- Weighing the pros and cons of protein
- Losing weight without dieting
- Understanding how supplements may do more harm than good
- Learning the truth about supplements
- Using coffee to boost energy and performance

Ask any bodybuilder, triathlete, or racehorse trainer about the importance of proper nutrition, and they're all likely to say the same thing: you are what you eat.

Sure, lifting can (and should) be an important part of your fitness regimen, but if you neglect proper nutrition, you're likely to sabotage your potential gains in the gym, as well as your overall health. We all know people who seem to flourish while eating a diet of pastrami sandwiches, jelly donuts, and milkshakes, but most people pay a steep price for such gluttony.

Typically, if you neglect your diet, you're destined to struggle with your weight, feel sluggish during the day, or, worse, invite sickness and disease. Even if you exercise regularly and have a washboard stomach, ignoring sound nutrition means you'll probably struggle through your workout. "I just didn't have it today" is a common complaint heard in the gym. It says a great deal about the individual's body chemistry and the lack of the fuel it needs to function.

As you probably know, enough myths and misinformation about nutrition are floating around to confuse even the most knowledgeable fitness aficionado. Don't despair. In this chapter, we walk you through this dietary quagmire and explain what constitutes a sensible diet. We also discuss the changes you may need to make as you improve your fitness level and health. If you have less body fat than an underfed marathoner, have more energy than a nuclear power plant, and eat plenty of fresh vegetables and lean protein, you probably should just skip to the next chapter. If not, grab a pen or pencil, and let's get shopping.

How Much Is Just Enough?

Let's start at the beginning—the basics of a sensible diet for the average healthy adult.

According to the U.S. Department of Agriculture (USDA), the "standard" reference male weighs 154 pounds, and his female counterpart tips the scales at 121. The phrases *Recommended Dietary Allowances (RDA)* and *Recommended Daily Intake (RDI)* refer to the levels of protein, vitamin, and mineral intake considered adequate to meet the nutritional needs of these exceedingly normal folks. Of course, if you weigh significantly more or less than those figures, you need to adjust accordingly. Similarly, if you're pregnant, lactating, postmenopausal, or a kid, your requirements differ from what the RDA suggests.

In 2011, the USDA unveiled the MyPlate icon, which replaced the Food Guide Pyramid. MyPlate emphasizes the fruit, vegetable, grains, protein, and dairy food groups.

A sixth group, the one that makes most of us salivate, is pleasing to the palate but high in fat and calories. This group includes fats, oils, and sweets. Sadly, these substances have little or no nutritive value and should be eaten sparingly. (One can only imagine the frenzy caused by a study stating that the best diet would include plentiful servings of ice cream, potato chips, mayonnaise, and bacon!)

Here's something else you should know: the six essential nutrients. They are as follows:

- Carbohydrates
- Proteins
- Fats
- Vitamins
- Minerals
- Water

FLEX FACTS

MyPlate provides a visual representation of a healthful diet. You can learn more at www.ChooseMyPlate.gov.

Before we get into the nuts and bolts of what and when to eat, let's do a quickie course in basic nutrition.

Carbohydrates (carbs), proteins, and fats are your sources of calories. Carbs supply 4 calories per gram and are classified as simple or complex. This isn't a psychological profile; it's based on the properties each possesses. Simple carbs, which are quickly converted to energy, are high in sugar and found in treats such as cakes, cookies, jams, and soda.

Complex carbohydrates, which provide a more sustained and gradual release of glucose into the bloodstream, are found in pasta, bread, grains, and cereals. Complex carbs should be the mainstay of your diet.

Fats don't provide a lot of vitamins and minerals, but they play a valuable role in your diet. For example, without ingesting some fat—about 2 tablespoons a day—your body couldn't process or absorb vitamins A, D, E, or K.

Protein, which forms the structural basis for muscle tissue, supplies energy only when not enough calories are available from carbs and fat. Foods high in protein include meat, milk, eggs, and legumes.

That's the basics on what we eat. Many experts disagree on the precise figures, but it's our informed opinion that a good diet should consist of 60 to 65 percent carbohydrates, 10 to 12 percent protein, and 20 to 30 percent fat. Here's a helpful key to figure out how much of each type of food you should eat.

First you need to figure out your basal metabolic rate (BMR). Your BMR is the amount of energy (calories) you'd burn just to keep going if you did nothing but lie in bed staring at the wall. (The ultimate couch potato doesn't even use the remote control.) It's both amusing and informative to figure out the approximate number of calories your body needs each day to maintain your weight. To figure out your BMR for one day, get your calculator and punch in the following numbers. This estimate should be within 15 percent of your actual BMR.

> Men: Body weight (pounds) $\times$ 24 $\div$ 2.2
>
> Women: Body weight (pounds) $\times$ 21 $\div$ 2.2

For example, Jonathan weighs 172 pounds. To find out his metabolic rate, he multiplies 172 by 24, which is 4,128; then he divides by 2.2 to get 1,876. So without exercising, he needs to consume 1,876 calories each day to maintain his body weight; thus, to lose weight, he needs to eat fewer than 1,876 calories. Now, Jonathan actually does more than lie prone for the day. In fact, he burns about 1,500 or so calories each day swimming, cycling, running, and lifting weights, which means he breaks even at more than 3,300 calories a day. (By way of comparison, the average sumo wrestler consumes 4,600 calories a day.) Being able to approximate your metabolic rate gives you an idea of how many calories your body needs each day.

Do You Need More?

As an aspiring body beautiful, you may be wondering whether your caloric needs are different than the average. Should you eat some extra protein? Maybe less fat? Good questions.

The Truth About Protein

When it comes to strength training and building muscle, the role of protein is perhaps the most misunderstood. First, some facts: the RDA for protein is 0.8 grams per kilogram. For our prototypical 154-pound (70-kilogram) friend, that's 56 grams of protein a day, or about 1 cup (9 grams) of milk, 2 eggs (12 grams), and a 4-ounce (32-gram) serving of chicken or beef. In other words, it's quite easy to meet the RDA requirement.

"Whoa, Nellie!" you may be saying. "You just said protein helps make up the actual structure of the muscle. If that's true, isn't it best to eat more protein?" At the risk of sounding like a politician on the campaign trail, the answer is "Yes and no."

Although scientific evidence suggests that some strength and endurance athletes may benefit from protein intakes of as much as 1.5 to 2.0 times the RDA, this is probably not necessary or helpful for the vast majority of people. The catch-22 is that you're probably already downing more than the RDA and just don't know it. So before you start doing a Rocky Balboa on us and slurping raw-egg shakes before heading to the gym, know that recent studies show the average American consumes more than 100 grams of protein per day. So although you may need more than the RDA, you're likely already there.

WEIGHT A MINUTE

Beware of "studies" that claim you should consume more than twice the amount of protein suggested by the RDA. Odds are, these are conducted by manufacturers of supplements who have a vested interest in your eating like a lion.

Water, Water, Everywhere

One of the most important things you can do to improve your performance is also one of the easiest. Simply ensure that you are adequately hydrated from the start to the conclusion of your workout. The body is about 60 percent water, and adequate hydration is essential to life, cellular homeostasis, joint function, and body temperature regulation, among other things.

According to Lauren Antonucci, a top sports nutritionist based in New York City, male athletes should consume 3.7 liters of fluid daily, while female athletes should aim for 2.7 liters daily. This is a good starting point and something most athletes can remember and easily track. Another relatively simple way for athletes to calculate their daily fluid needs is to drink half their body weight in fluid ounces (so, for example, a 160-pound athlete would drink 80 ounces of fluid, and a 130-pound athlete would drink 65 ounces) *plus* an additional 24 to 32 ounces per hour of activity after the first hour. Of course, this should serve as a starting point. Individual needs vary widely, and environmental conditions (heat, humidity, and elevation) must also be taken into account.

Furthermore, athletes should ensure that they drink 5 to 7 mL/kg of body weight (2 to 3 milliliters per pound of body weight), or about 8 to 16 ounces for the average athlete, 2 to 3 hours before beginning their exercise, to allow for optimal hydration and excretion of excess fluid intake before exercise commences. During exercise, athletes should aim to replace as much of the fluid they lose to sweat as possible, ideally to minimize water deficit to less than 2 percent of total body weight (for example, a weight loss of no more than 3 pounds for a 150-pound athlete). Clearly, sweat rates vary widely by individual and environmental conditions, and can range from 0.5 liters to 2.5 liters of water per hour. Antonucci recommends conducting periodic "sweat tests" during practice to determine your individual sweat rate. Weigh yourself before and after exercise. If you weigh less afterward, you're sweating at a faster rate than you're replacing the fluids and you need to drink a little more. Remember, 1 pound of body weight is equivalent to 16 ounces of water.

Many exercisers fail to consume adequate fluids following exercise and would be well served by following a fluid-replacement plan that includes 16 to 24 ounces of fluid for each pound lost to sweat during exercise. Drinking a beverage that contains sodium or drinking water along with sodium-containing foods best helps replace both fluid and electrolyte needs and improves recovery.

SPOT ME

During exercise, don't wait until you're thirsty to start drinking. By the time you're thirsty, you're already well on your way to becoming dehydrated.

Consider some salient facts about water:

- Water is responsible for providing the building materials for cell protoplasm. Don't ask—just trust us: it's important.

- Water helps protect the body's tissue and internal organs.

- Water helps regulate body temperature, as well as transport other nutrients, hormones, and waste products.

There's more, but we assume that you get the point by now: the more water you drink, the better you'll feel.

The Fancy Stuff

Okay, so water is cool, but what about Gatorade, Sportsade, and the scores of other liquid "ades" sprouting up all over the beverage aisle? After all, if it works for Michael Jordan, it's got to be good, right? To which we reply unequivocally, "Maybe." Unless you're running, cycling, or engaging in any cardiovascular activity for at least 45 minutes to an hour a day or working out in a hot, humid gym, sports drinks really aren't necessary. Your body has no real physiological need for the extra calories or minerals in a sports drink. (You'll replenish everything you need at your next meal.)

FLEX FACTS

In the 1960s, a fluid-replacement drink was developed at the University of Florida for the school's athletic teams, which train and play in hot, muggy weather nearly all year long. It was called Gatorade, after the Gators, the nickname of all the school's teams. Gatorade contains some vitamins and minerals, but it's mostly sugar and water.

However, if you are pounding the pavement with a vengeance, a sports drink may help you speed up the rate at which your body absorbs the fluid. Perhaps the biggest advantage these sporty drinks have over straight water is taste. A cold glass of pure mountain water may be the elixir of life, but after a while, your taste buds may be calling out for more. Simply put, the more you like the taste, the more likely you are to drink the stuff.

Here are our top three tips for optimal hydration:

- Most commercial sports drinks contain a carbohydrate concentration of between 5 and 7 percent. Anything higher than that can cause gastric distress and actually slow fluid absorption. Diluted juice (50 percent juice/50 percent water) with maybe a pinch of salt works just as well.

- Drink 16 ounces of cold water or diluted sports drink before working out.

- Drink water every 15 minutes or so to prevent dehydration.

Lose It by the Book

We are a culture obsessed with weight, for two reasons. First, we have before us the unrealistic standards set by the incredibly thin supermodels and actors who are viewed as "ideal." Second, we are the most overweight culture in the Western world. And oddly enough, despite our nation's keen interest in fitness, the obesity rates are on the rise.

If you're one of the millions of Americans struggling to lose weight, you're well aware of the countless products and diets promising to help you "drop those ugly pounds" in a matter of minutes (okay, days). Not only are most of these products bogus, dangerous, or worse, but even the best of them rarely produce long-term weight loss.

Slow but Steady Wins the Race

With few exceptions, following very-low-calorie diets, skipping meals, and fasting are counterproductive. When you make drastic adjustments to your caloric intake, your body's survival instincts sound an alarm and slow your metabolism to a snail's pace. Your goal is to speed up your metabolic rate, not the other way around. When you sit down to your next meal after a fast, your metabolism remains depressed, which actually causes you to gain weight.

Because most health experts agree that a weight loss of more than 2 pounds per week is unhealthy, we recommend a weekly goal of 1 pound. Usually, when you lose more than that per week, you're actually losing muscle as well as fat—a big no-no. Not only does muscle look good, but it also helps you burn calories.

To lose 1 pound a week, you need to burn 500 calories more than you ingest each day. That may seem like a formidable number, but it really isn't if you exercise. If you can manage to burn an extra 250 calories a day—a 2.5-mile jog or 30 minutes on the exercise bike—you're halfway there. Remember, your body won't know whether you get those miles walking to the post office or running in the park. Also keep in mind that as you increase your muscle mass, you burn extra calories. Even as you read this book, your muscles are metabolically active. (Reading this book while you walk to the post office is even better.)

Here are some handy ways to decrease the number of calories you eat each day:

- In the morning, eat a piece of whole-wheat toast instead of a bagel. *Calories saved:* 150.

- Hold the mayo and use mustard on your turkey sandwich. *Calories saved:* 100.

- Use tomato sauce (without sugar) instead of a creamy alfredo on your pasta. *Calories saved:* 190.

- Use skim or low-fat soy milk in place of whole milk. *Calories saved:* 60.

- Pass on the midday candy bar and down a piece of fruit. *Calories saved:* 180. (If you're still hungry, eat raw nuts.)

- Toss that can of cola and drink water. *Calories saved:* 150.

- Use one instead of two sugars in your coffee. Better yet, use none. Calories saved: 15 to 30.

FLEX FACTS

Men with more than 25 percent body fat and women with more than 30 percent body fat are considered obese. Studies by the National Center of Health Statistics over the last two decades show that today approximately 35 percent of women and 31 percent of men age 20 and older are considered obese. That's an increase of approximately 30 percent and 25 percent, respectively, from 1980.

The Sad Truth About Fad Diets

As P. T. Barnum might have said, "A weight-loss sucker is born every minute." No matter how outrageous or absurd the alternative, many people refuse to apply common sense and sound science to their dietary needs (or their pocketbooks). Recently, we heard a radio spot for a product called The Fat Assassin that promised to melt off pounds quicker than you can spell John Wilkes Booth. Although the image is clearly preposterous, enough people are apparently buying it to justify the number of ads on the air.

You can learn the hard way or take our word for it right now: wacky diets such as the Grapefruit Diet or the Cabbage Diet that exclude or severely restrict whole categories of food do more harm than good because they typically exclude important vitamins and minerals.

Take Barry Sears's The Zone, a low-carbohydrate diet that in the 1990s gained more notoriety than Monica Lewinsky. A few years ago, one of the guys Jonathan trains with raved about how he'd lost 7 pounds in just a week by following Sears's 40-30-30 diet (40 percent of your daily calories from carbohydrates, 30 percent from protein, and 30 percent from fat). Basically, the premise of The Zone diet is that eating too many carbs makes you fat.

Jonathan, who seemingly gets joy from telling little children there's no Santa Claus, was more than happy to point out the flaw in The Zone theory. True, his training buddy had lost a whopping 7 pounds in seven days; however, when you know that carbs, which are stored in the body as glycogen, hold three times their weight in water, you realize that this suddenly svelte Zone-ite had lost water and sugar, not fat. That's a good way to travel if you're like Deidre trying to make weight for a powerlifting competition, but it's useless if your aim is to drop fat. Once again, if something seems too good to be true, it probably is. In most cases, long-term weight loss from low-carbohydrate diets comes from the fact that the diets are also low in calories—not because they're low in carbs.

FLEX FACTS

Elite male marathoners generally carry about 4 to 6 percent body fat. Football linemen can range from 17 to 23 percent. When Deidre won her first World Powerlifting title, she carried 14 percent body fat. Essential body fat, the amount necessary for normal physiologic function, is approximately 3 percent in men and 12 percent in women. These levels may interfere with normal function and are not necessary for optimal health. Males at 15 to 18 percent and females at 19 to 23 percent body fat are considered healthy.

A Pound of Feathers or a Pound of Rocks

As we've mentioned, the scale doesn't know the difference between 1 pound of water and 1 pound of fat. The same can be said about the difference between muscle and fat. Plainly put, "A pound is a pound is a pound" on the scale. However, there's actually a huge difference between the way a pound of muscle and a pound of fat look on the human body.

When clients tell Jonathan they're frustrated that they haven't lost weight despite their best efforts, he reminds them that they've dropped a dress size or a belt loop. The bottom line isn't what the scale says, but your ratio of fat to lean mass.

For example, consider two chaps who stand 5 feet, 10 inches and tip the scales at 180 pounds. Mr. Stud Muffin has only 10 percent (or 18 pounds) of body fat, while Mr. Potato Latke is schlepping 25 percent of his weight as fat. That means Mr. Latke has more than twice the fat of his counterpart. The scale can't tell them apart, but a measurement of their body fat sure can.

You can gauge your percentage of body fat in many ways—underwater weighing is the most accurate, but most knowledgeable trainers with skin-fold calipers can give you a reasonable assessment. However, the best way to see where you stand is to step in front of a mirror in the buff and look for yourself.

To Supplement or Not?

If you think that eating right is a challenge, a trip through your local vitamin shop can be downright treacherous. Let's take a look at what supplements help you meet your fitness goals and which ones not only fail to help and waste your money, but may actually harm you.

Buyer Beware

First of all, the most common dietary deficiencies are carbohydrates and fluids—neither of which requires a trip to a health food store. Second, vitamin, protein, and mineral deficiencies are rare in people with a balanced diet. You should also know that although a shortage of a nutrient can have a negative effect, taking an excess of one particular substance usually does more harm than good. For instance, a protein deficiency can leave you feeling sluggish, but ingesting excess protein can actually cause weight gain and kidney problems.

In 1989, the Food and Drug Administration (FDA) defined a dietary supplement as a substance made of essential nutrients such as vitamins, minerals, and amino acids. The following year, an act of legislation came down the pike broadening the term *dietary supplements* to include herbs and similar nutritional substances. Then in 1994, another act from the feds established yet another definition. Here are the rules that allow a company to identify and market a product as a dietary supplement today:

- The product must be labeled as a "dietary supplement."

- The product must contain one or more of the following ingredients: vitamin, mineral, herb or other botanical, and amino acids. (There are other criteria, but they're too tedious to mention.)

- The product is intended for ingestion in pill, capsule, tablet, or liquid form. In other words, desiccated caterpillars from China fall outside the guidelines.

- The product must not be represented as a conventional food or as the sole item of a meal or diet. The Complete One-Pill Breakfast, Lunch, or Dinner ain't cuttin' it right now.

It's worth noting that these regulations require the manufacturer's statements to be "truthful and not misleading" but do not establish any standard for the often outrageous claims that supposedly back up such statements. In other words, a single study—even one financed by the manufacturer using shaky statistical methods—is enough, even if that one study contradicts scores of other, more impartial studies. And you wonder how Jonathan became such a skeptic.

When you're browsing the aisles in your local health food store, study the fine print on the product's label. If you see "This statement has not been evaluated by the FDA," you should think, "Buyer beware." Claims made on food labels are more strictly regulated than on supplement labels and, hence, must answer to a higher authority.

Before we get into some of the most popular individual supplements on the market, consider these random facts on dietary supplements:

- Supplements include vitamins and minerals, as well as herbals and botanicals.

- Multivitamins may help some people, but less is known about herbals and botanicals.

- High doses of certain supplements may be harmful.

- Don't assume that *natural* means "safe." The two words are not synonymous. Tobacco is natural, and we know the often lethal long-term risks of using that product.

- If you want to ensure that you're getting all you need, eat a variety of foods.

Powder Power

Earlier in this chapter, we discussed how most people get more than enough protein in their diet. However, occasionally vegetarians or folks on low-calorie diets may be protein deficient. Even if you fall into that category, there's no reason to run out and buy a tub of the Super Mega Muscle Man Protein Powder you may have seen advertised in a fitness magazine.

In grad school, Jonathan had occasion to examine such a powder. The label of this "miracle" mix of muscle-building powder purported to have the ideal combination of amino acids, which are the building blocks of protein. According to the directions, the optimal way to use the powder was to mix it with a glass of skim milk. However, on closer inspection, Jonathan and his classmates determined that at least one third of the amino acids in this miraculous concoction came from the skim milk. Considering that the powder cost a few bucks per serving and the milk retailed for roughly 20¢, all you had to do was down three glasses of skim milk, and you'd have achieved the same effect. If you're totally sold on powders, try evaporated nonfat dry milk. Antidairy? Soy milk or rice milk should fit the bill.

WEIGHT A MINUTE

Don't believe everything you read. Many of the manufacturers of the supplements advertised in some of the most popular "muscle" and fitness magazines own the magazine their products appear in. If that's the case, don't expect an unbiased opinion of a product.

Starbucks, Anyone?

In the "old" days, you could get a good cup of coffee in New York City for 50¢. Today, in the era of gourmet coffee shops, half a buck gets you into the men's room. Simply put, coffee has become big business. While you can drop $3.50 for a mocha latte cappuccino at Starbucks, caffeine—a substance banned by the International Olympic Committee—is one of the cheapest and perhaps most beneficial ergogenic aids out there. (Just for the record: to get booted from the Olympics for abusing caffeine, you'd have to top out way above the dose that is allowable and most beneficial.)

Caffeine helps you in two ways. During aerobic activities, it can increase the availability of fat as fuel. And although it won't make you stronger during weightlifting, some evidence shows that caffeine helps make the activity seem easier.

Before you start swilling shots of espresso, keep the following in mind:

- Caffeine can cause gastrointestinal problems.

- Drinking too much can make you jittery.

- Caffeine is a diuretic. Drink extra water if you're going to work up a sweat.

- Possible links exist between caffeine consumption and benign fibrocystic breast disease.

- If you have an ulcer or irregular heartbeat, your best bet is to stick to decaf.

WEIGHT A MINUTE

HMB (hydroxymethylbutyrate), creatine, pyruvate, inosine, branch-chained amino acids, bee pollen, and ginseng are supplements you might have heard about. None of them impress us, for a variety of reasons, mainly because we're concerned about whether they're safe and effective.

The Bar Scene

Flip through any bicycle or runner's apparel catalogue, and you're bound to see a host of ads for energy bars such as PowerBar, Clif Bar, Met-Rx Bar, Balance Bar, PR Ironman Bar … and the list goes on. Each makes bold claims about what it can do for you, from optimizing your body's natural ability to burn stored fat for energy, to providing you with a burst of energy. Not only are they supposed to start your engine and keep it running at optimal efficiency, but they're designed to taste good (unlike their ancestors, which tasted a tad better than the rubber flooring in your gym). Check out some of these flavors: white chocolate mocha, berry blast, cookie dough, and Kona crunch. Sounds like a get-together at a Ben & Jerry's convention.

These smartly marketed products are good under a variety of conditions, including when you're doing a long training ride, when you're too hungry to work out but too busy to eat, and when you need a late-night snack but a piece of fruit just doesn't have enough oomph. Most of these bars are easily digested and pack a fair number of nutrients in a convenient package. When Jonathan wakes up at the obscene hour of 5 A.M. for a bike race, he's usually too comatose to prepare breakfast and simply downs a PowerBar as a prerace meal.

Consider a few energy bar tidbits:

- Most bars are fairly high in carbohydrates, which are more readily digested than calories from protein or fat.

- Some, however, are extremely high in protein and may not be easy to digest. As we've said, extra protein often does more harm than good.

- Beware of bars that make outrageous claims. These bars are a good source of food to help stabilize blood sugar levels and fight hunger pangs, but they're not going to make you burn fat faster. And they're not going to make you stronger or faster. Despite what he and the advertisers may say, six-time Ironman Triathlon winner Mark Allen didn't run down his competition because he ate PR Bars. (In fact, given his talent and training regimen, he could have eaten a bar of soap and still dominated.)

From A to Zinc

One of the most interesting facts about vitamin and mineral supplementation is that, more often than not, if you believe that taking them is good for you, it is. In other words, the power of the mind to invest positive qualities in things we believe are good for us is not to be denied. (Studies on the placebo effect are nothing short of remarkable: patients with inoperative cancer who were given a "miracle" cure [sugar pills] actually saw their cancer temporarily go into remission.)

That said, both competitive and recreational athletes tend to overdose on vitamins and minerals, considering that most people who eat a balanced diet get more than enough from the foods they eat. However, the most common vitamins missing in our diets are B_6, B_{12} (typically found in animal products), E (found in vegetable oils), and folic acid (found in leafy green vegetables and organ meats). In addition, many women don't get enough calcium and iron in their diet.

Megadosing on vitamins is probably a waste of time and money—and, in the case of fat-soluble vitamins and minerals, detrimental—but taking a multivitamin can be a safe, inexpensive insurance policy against deficiencies caused by poor diet.

The Least You Need to Know

- Sound nutrition starts with sound science.
- When it comes to building muscle, protein is the most misunderstood food group.
- Proper hydration is crucial, but sports drinks have their place in the diets of serious athletes.
- Eschew fad diets and practice the only real way to lose weight: moderation, variety, and balance.
- The scale doesn't lie, but it doesn't tell the whole truth, either. Your percentage of body fat is just as important as how much you weigh.
- Nutritional supplements are big business. Read the labels and beware of outrageous claims.

Getting a Clean Bill of Health

In This Chapter

- Understanding the importance of a medical checkup
- Heeding medical precautions and prescriptions
- Handling injuries
- Learning the medical benefits of weight training
- Practicing safety
- Making your way around the gym
- Playing nice: courtesy counts in the gym

Here's an amusing paradox: when you're sick or injured, it's nearly impossible to think or talk about anything other than your health or lack of it. When Joe broke his wrist before his kayaking season a while back, he had to muzzle himself not to mention it to perfect strangers. "Excuse me, sir, I've broken one of my carpal bones. Care to hear this gripping tale?" Conversely, there's almost nothing more tedious on Earth than listening to someone tell you about his or her health problems—unless, of course, you have the same condition. In fact, put three guys with broken wrists in a room together and provide refreshments, and they'll entertain themselves till the bones heal.

We note this phenomenon because of the importance of consulting with your physician before you head to the gym, and knowing what you need to be aware of—medically speaking—when you embark on a new exercise regimen. Given its clinical nature, this section may seem a bit on the dry side. On the other hand, we offer you some important information about how to keep yourself healthy and strong while working out to get even healthier and stronger. If it's been a while since you've had a checkup or exercised on a regular basis, or if you've had (or have) a serious medical condition, you need to take special care. But there's good news: very few people need to be excluded from working out—although modifications may be necessary. Read on for more info.

The Medical Checkup

The prudent path to follow when you're starting a weightlifting regimen is to see your doctor for a thorough checkup. Again, this is especially important if you've been inactive for a while, have a bad back, are overweight, or are over 45. To some, getting a checkup is an odious task. Assuming that your doctor is decent, it shouldn't be. In health and fitness (as in virtually anything else), knowledge is power. Think of getting a physical not as a burden, but as an opportunity to become more powerful. Okay, let's say that you haven't been sick in 10 years, you're 29 years old, and the idea of visiting a doctor is as appealing as having a root canal. The generally accepted minimal standard to gauge whether you're ready to work out is a seven-question self-evaluation called the Physical Activity Readiness Questionnaire (PAR-Q). Designed for people between the ages of 15 and 69, it was developed by the Canadian Society for Exercise Physiology to see whether you've got the mettle to push some metal.

PAR-Q and YOU
(A Questionnaire for People Aged 15 to 69)

Regular physical activity is fun and healthy, and more people are starting to become increasingly active every day. Being more active is very safe for most people. However, some people should check with their doctor before they start becoming physically active.

If you are planning to become much more physically active than you are now, start by answering the seven questions below. If you are between the ages of 15 and 69, the PAR-Q will tell you if you should check with your doctor before you start. If you are over 69 years of age, and you are not used to being very active, check with your doctor.

Common sense is your best guide when you answer these questions. Please read the questions carefully and answer each one honestly: check YES or NO.

Yes	No	
❑	❑	1. Has your doctor ever said that you have a heart condition and that you should only do physical activity recommended by a doctor?
❑	❑	2. Do you feel pain in your chest when you do physical activity?
❑	❑	3. In the past month, have you had chest pain when you were not doing physical activity?
❑	❑	4. Do you lose your balance because of dizziness, or do you ever lose consciousness?
❑	❑	5. Do you have a bone or joint problem that could be made worse by a change in your physical activity?
❑	❑	6. Is your doctor currently prescribing drugs (for example, water pills) for your blood pressure or heart condition?
❑	❑	7. Do you know of any other reason why you should not do physical activity?

If you answered …

YES to one or more questions

Talk with your doctor by phone or in person BEFORE you start to become much more physically active or before you have a fitness appraisal. Tell your doctor about the PAR-Q and which questions you answered YES.

- You may be able to do any activity you want—as long as you start slowly and build up gradually. Or, you may need to restrict your activities to those that are safe for you. Talk with your doctor about the kinds of activities you wish to participate in and follow his/her advice.

- Find out which community programs are safe and helpful for you.

NO to all questions

If you answered NO to *all* PAR-Q questions, you can be reasonably sure that you can:

- Start becoming much more physically active—begin slowly and build up gradually. This is the safest and easiest way to go.

- Take part in a fitness appraisal—this is an excellent way to determine your basic fitness so that you can plan the best way for you to live actively.

DELAY BECOMING MUCH MORE ACTIVE …

- If you are not feeling well because of a temporary illness such as a cold or a fever—wait until you feel better; or

- If you are or may be pregnant—talk to your doctor before you start becoming more active.

Please note: if your health changes so that you then answer YES to any of the above questions, tell your fitness or health professional. Ask whether you should change your physical activity plan.

Informed use of the PAR-Q: The Canadian Society for Exercise Physiology, Health Canada, and their agents assume no liability for persons who undertake physical activity, and if in doubt after completing this questionnaire, consult your doctor prior to physical activity.

If you answered "Yes" to any of these questions, or if you're older than 69, head straight to your doctor's office and tell the doctor that you responded affirmatively to one of the questions on the Physical Activity Readiness Questionnaire. Then let him or her give you a good once-over.

On the other hand, if you honestly answered "No" to these probing questions, the PAR-Q says it's okay to go ahead and have at it—but only if you do so gradually and follow all the safety precautions we outline for you throughout the book. (Just to put our prudent approach in perspective, even if you're in tremendous physical condition, it's unwise to start a new regimen like a lifter possessed. Starting out too fast is a sure way to get injured, even if you're fit.)

Most people over the age of 50 or so are concerned about heart disease, and for good reason. Heart attacks and strokes remain the single biggest killers in the United States. Because exercising puts extra strain on your heart and blood vessels, you need to be especially sure that your cardiovascular system is in good working order. Here are the risk factors for coronary artery disease set forth by the American College of Sports Medicine. See where you stack up under any of the following categories:

- **Age.** At greatest risk are men over the age of 45; women at greatest risk are those over 55 and those who experienced premature menopause without estrogen replacement therapy.

- **A family history of heart attacks or strokes.** Sudden death of your father (or another close male relative) before the age of 55 or your mother (or close female relative) before the age of 65 is a risk factor. Genes are powerful, so don't stick your head in the sand if your family's history is sketchy. Get checked out.

- **Cigarette smoking.** Anyone who can read knows that smoking contributes to lung cancer, heart disease, and a host of other physical problems. We'll spare you the lecture, but if you smoke and want to work out, see your doctor before you launch a fitness regimen. Of course, it's better to work out and smoke than to just smoke, but our guess is that the more you get into the gym, the less you'll suck the cigarettes.

- **Hypertension.** Exercise is one of the best antidotes for this condition and often cures the condition without the need for medication. However, you need to be sure you're not stressing an already stressed-out circulatory system. See your doc if you've got any doubts.

- **High cholesterol.** Volumes have been written about good and bad cholesterol—what's high, what's low, what's dangerous, and what's not. Your doctor can tell you what's best for you, but a good rule of thumb is that you're considered at risk if your total cholesterol is more than 200 mg/dL or if your HDL (or "good cholesterol") is below 35 mg/dL. (For the record, mg/dL is the abbreviation for milligrams per deciliter.) Again, exercise has a beneficial effect in increasing your HDL, but be sure that you're not an egg yolk away from doing yourself serious harm.

- **Diabetes mellitus.** The connection between diabetes and heart disease is well known, so if you've been insulin dependent for more than 15 years or are over age 30 with diabetes, you're considered at risk. The same is true of non–insulin-dependent diabetics over 35.

- **Physical inactivity.** If your job keeps you pasted to your seat most of the day, or if the most arduous thing you've done in a year or more is play badminton at the company picnic, you're considered at risk if you engage in strenuous physical activity.

These risk factors don't mean that you shouldn't or can't work out, but you should exercise a little extra caution before you get started. And the first step you take should be to the doctor's office.

> **FLEX FACTS**
>
> A "normal" healthy blood pressure is around 120/80. Hypertension, or high blood pressure, is defined as any reading of 140/90 or more. By definition, blood pressure is the pressure exerted on the wall of a blood vessel. The first number, systolic pressure, occurs as the heart contracts; while the second number, diastolic pressure, occurs when the heart relaxes between beats.

"The Doctor Will See You Now"

Weight training can help treat a variety of ailments, especially if it's combined with a good stretching program and sound nutrition. We're not going to be so bold as to say that weight training can cure serious maladies like beriberi or foot-and-mouth disease, but it often does wonders for an ailing body. Having said that, weightlifting will exacerbate a number of conditions if you lift without medical supervision.

We don't mean to dampen your enthusiasm or frighten you off the exercise train; in fact, that's the last thing we want to do—well, the second to the last. We're most eager to help you avoid injuries or aggravate a preexisting condition. It may seem obvious, but we mention it anyway: when you're having a checkup, be sure to bring up any current problems you're experiencing. In other words, don't try to turn the doctor into a mind reader. After you've had your physical and learned how to safely proceed, find out if the gym you belong to (or are thinking about joining) has trainers who know how to work around your particular condition. Working with a trainer who isn't adept at handling stroke victims or heart patients—if that's your problem—is a big mistake.

Avoiding Risky Business

Okay, so you have high blood pressure or some other medical condition that provides a convenient excuse not to work out. Know this: 90 percent of the physical restrictions people live with are self-imposed. A few years back, a man with AIDS ran, cycled, and swam across the United States to prove to himself (and others) that people with this life-threatening disease can do far more than anyone realized. Just to drive home the point further: a man paralyzed from the waist down climbed Yosemite's El Capitan, one of the grandest rock faces in the world. Triathletes with missing limbs compete on a regular basis, as do athletes who have had organ transplants, strokes, and other medical challenges.

Let's look at some of the more common afflictions people have to deal with as they pertain to working out.

Hyper Types

Hypertension, or high blood pressure, is a condition that affects millions of Americans by placing chronic, increased stress on the normal function of the cardiovascular system. Often called the silent killer, hypertension is particularly insidious because it often goes undetected until you see the doctor or even have a heart attack or stroke.

Deidre has a photo taken of her deadlifting 365 pounds during a powerlifting competition. What's striking about it, besides the fact that she's lifting the equivalent of a baby elephant, is the terrific strain that shows on her face: her eyes bulge like Marty Feldman's, and the veins in her neck are engorged like bloated worms. (We call this the Beauty and the Beast syndrome.) Few of us are likely to try to hoist triple our body weight, but the fact remains that weightlifting can increase your blood pressure during the actual exercise.

A common mistake is holding your breath while lifting. We talk more about this once we get you into the gym, but for now, it's worth mentioning that holding your breath is ill advised—with high blood pressure or without. Competitive lifters like Deidre often hold their breath when they're shooting for a personal record (PR), but doing so may cause you bodily harm.

> **WEIGHT A MINUTE**
>
> Holding your breath while lifting causes an exaggerated and sometimes dangerously high increase in blood pressure. The technical term for holding your breath during a lift is a Valsalva maneuver.

Post-Stroke Fitness

For some stroke victims, embarking on a weightlifting program can be an essential part of their recovery. For others, doing so can be downright dangerous. If you've had a stroke, you need to discuss weight training with your doctor to see which category of patient you are.

Typically, if one side of your body is impaired or severely restricted, a knowledgeable physical therapist or trainer will have you work a lot on your unaffected side because this part of your body will now be working much harder to compensate.

Deidre, who has worked for two decades as a physical therapist, has done a lot of work with stroke victims and is continually amazed by the progress people are able to make. One of her most remarkable patients is a woman in her 80s who had a stroke 12 years ago. She was unable to use her right arm and walked with the use of a brace on her right leg and a cane. Even so, she walked outside alone every day and was able to cook and clean for herself.

Post-Heart Attack Workout

For some, a heart attack spells the beginning of the end. Victims sense their own mortality and just "try to take it easy," which does little except make them sluggish and more prone to poor health. For others, surviving heart disease is like a second lease on life and a chance to nurture health instead of abuse it or take it for granted.

If you've had a heart attack or are at high risk for one, your doctor may well recommend that you join a cardiac rehabilitation program—which has strict guidelines for cardiovascular as well as strength-training exercise—or simply encourage you to start exercising slowly. In the latter case, it's wise to work with a trainer or physical therapist who specializes in cardiac rehab. Combining aerobic activity, which can strengthen your heart (which is, after all, a muscle), and a sound diet will no doubt change your life.

Breathing Right

Asthma is a nasty affliction, with symptoms that include wheezing, chest congestion, chest tightness, coughing, and shortness of breath. Exercising in cold, dry air is usually the most troublesome for asthmatics; activities such as swimming are often tolerated much better. Thoroughly warming up before exercising can help prevent symptoms, and many athletes with asthma have risen to the top of their game. Just look at former marathon world record holder Alberto Salazar or Olympic gold medalist Jackie Joyner-Kersee, who have both been diagnosed with asthma. Jonathan also was severely afflicted with asthma as a child but nevertheless may be the best athlete in his apartment building. (Actually, Jonathan has benefited greatly from exercise, and although he never trains without his inhaler, his condition no longer prevents him from competing.)

FLEX FACTS

During the 1992 Summer Olympics, many television viewers were shocked to find out that track-and-field champion Jackie Joyner-Kersee suffers from asthma. Joyner-Kersee is perhaps the greatest woman athlete ever, and her performance proved that asthma does not necessarily prevent exercise, even given the demands of top-level competition.

Today, with advances in medications that can help prevent or alleviate symptoms with few side effects, asthmatics have every reason to exercise if they so choose. Your doctor can prescribe an inhaler to help; keep it with you whenever you're exercising, in case symptoms arise.

The Sugar Blues

Diabetes is a disease in which the body produces an insufficient amount of insulin (a hormone necessary for the metabolism of blood glucose or blood sugar). This leads to an abnormally high blood glucose level. When the body functions normally, it releases insulin to counteract the increased sugar as blood glucose levels rise after eating. In diabetics, either the body does not release enough insulin (as in the case of Type I, juvenile-onset diabetes) or the body is insulin resistant, in which case insulin doesn't do what it's supposed to (as in the more common Type II, adult-onset diabetes). If the blood sugar level dips, extreme hunger pangs and dizziness result. If it's bad enough, blackouts and/or diabetic shock follow.

Because some exercise can have an "insulinlike" effect, sometimes insulin dosages need to be altered after you begin an exercise program. Furthermore, you might have to change the site where you inject the insulin: injecting into a working muscle may increase the rate at which the body absorbs the insulin.

Changes in your diet can cure or drastically improve adult-onset diabetes. If you do regulate your diabetes this way, be sure you eat before working out. Talk to your doctor or a nutritionist about the best time to structure your workouts so that they coincide with your normal blood sugar levels.

Building Bones

Years ago, lifting weights was considered "unladylike." Now medical science has come around to tell us that taking to the gym is an effective way for postmenopausal women to combat osteoporosis, a disease that causes the loss of bone density. A proper diet that includes plenty of calcium and magnesium and a gradual weight-training program can work wonders to prevent the disease from developing. Once osteoporosis has set in, however, it's important for you to get clearance from your doctor that you can safely lift weights.

Bum Knees

A seemingly endless number of things can cause your knees to ache—from running, to using poor posture, to ballroom dancing. Sometimes postural awareness can cure your knees; sometimes a stretching program can alleviate your pain. If you pursue those remedies and your knees still ache, have your doctor check them. When you get the go-ahead, go easy. Often strengthening the muscles in your quadriceps and hamstrings will ease your pain.

Oy, My Back

Back pain is one of the most complicated issues in the medical profession. Your back is made of literally hundreds of bones, muscles, ligaments, and nerves—any of which can go on the fritz, depending on what you're doing and the amount of stress you're under. Consult a doctor if you're experiencing serious trouble. One key to preventing back pain is maintaining strength and flexibility in your "core" muscles. We discuss that later, in Chapter 12.

Atlas Shrugged

The shoulder is an amazing joint. Maybe the credit belongs to our simian ancestors, who swung through the trees with the greatest of ease. Regardless, the range of motion the shoulder provides the arm is just short of miraculous. Think of a swimmer doing windmills to warm up for a race, or think back to the last time you threw a Hail Mary pass in a touch football game.

But because the shoulder is so mobile and flexible, it's also prone to injury. Shoulder injuries are one of the most common maladies caused by weightlifting—generally from lifting too much weight with too little form. Weightlifting can also aggravate an existing minor injury.

The two "itises"—*tendonitis* and *bursitis*—and rotator cuff tears are common injuries brought on by repetitive activity such as playing racket sports and swimming. They all result in the same symptom: shoulder pain. It's normal for your shoulders to feel sore after serious exertion, like helping your cousin Ruth move to a fourth-floor walk-up or playing a game of ultimate Frisbee. But if it's been business as usual and you experience shoulder pain at rest or with movement, see your doctor.

DEFINITION

Anything that ends in *itis* means inflammation. **Tendonitis** is an inflammation of the tendons (the connective tissue that connects bone to muscle), and **bursitis** is an inflammation of the bursa (padlike sacs found between tendons and bones that act to reduce friction).

Under the Weather

One last bit of advice on a common question about the merits of working out when you're not feeling well. Ready for this political answer? Sometimes it can help, and sometimes it can hurt. Generally, if all you have is a cold and all your symptoms are above your neck (sniffles, a tickly throat, and so on), a moderate workout can help clear your head. If your symptoms have spread to your chest or include a fever or body aches, working out is likely to worsen the condition. In that case, we recommend that you rest, recover, and have at it when you're feeling better.

Safety in the Gym

Just because you've gotten the all-clear from your doctor doesn't mean you're free of danger. In fact, the gym can be a treacherous place. After finishing several sets on the bench press years ago, Joe and a friend were removing 45-pound *plates* from either side of the barbell. Protocol dictates that each person remove the plates more or less at the same time. Joe, however, wasn't paying attention and removed all the weight from his end before his friend grabbed his side. The weighted side made like a seesaw, and the plate fell smack on his friend's big toe. Later they had a good laugh about "Crack-a-toe-a," but at the time, Joe's momentary lapse left his friend hobbled for weeks.

DEFINITION

Plates are what you add to each side of a bar to increase its weight. Plates you'll see in most gyms come in denominations of 2½, 5, 10, 25, 35, and 45 pounds.

Understanding safety issues in the gym is extremely important. People do get injured in health clubs, and usually the injury was avoidable. Jonathan has lost count of the number of times he's had to sprint from one end of the gym to the other to pull a bar off the chest of a beefy dude who thought a spotter was reserved for the scrawny types.

There aren't a lot of gym safety rules, and they're not terribly complicated, but they are specific to this unique environment where motivated individuals (many of whom are wearing headphones) are hoisting large metal objects overhead.

Let's take a look at proper gym etiquette, correct form, and common safety concerns, such as being sure the barbell collars are in place, being mindful of where you drop your weights, and knowing the right way to "spot" for someone. The key is consideration and awareness. If you were in danger of hurting only yourself, that would be one thing, but you become a threat to others if you start turning toes into pancakes on a regular basis.

Form, Form (and Form)

Hang out in a gym long enough, and you'll hear a litany of complaints—injured shoulders, stiff backs, tweaked biceps, and strained hamstrings. The causes are many and varied, but the biggest culprit is bad technique. Proper technique is the key not only to making solid strength gains, but also to maintaining health over the long term.

Generally, using good form means lifting *less* weight than you might think you're able to. Proper form requires you to isolate the muscle or muscles you're trying to build, which makes the exercise harder to perform.

We give you a complete description of the proper way to execute each exercise we recommend in the appropriate chapters, but keep in mind that the actual amount of weight you lift is, in many ways, insignificant. Instead, what's important is how you lift that weight. Remember that you're lifting to improve your body and mind, not to pump up your ego. Lifting slowly through a full range of motion is your ultimate goal. If you practice proper technique from the beginning, you'll build a solid base—strength from the inside out. Slow, controlled movements and proper breathing are a few of the key components we stress.

SPOT ME

By practicing proper form, you maximize the benefits of lifting while minimizing the danger. Never try to squeeze out an extra rep at the expense of form or safety.

What Goes Where?

The first time you walk into a gym, you might feel like a city slicker dropped off in the middle of a forest. The texture of the landscape is so foreign that you might feel dizzy with anxiety and confusion. But don't feel bad: to the uninitiated, the gym is a jungle, and you don't know where anything goes or what any of these shiny metal contraptions do.

Fret not! After you learn the lay of the land, you'll waltz through the establishment like a deer bounding through the woods. In the following section, we discuss the typical layout of most gyms, where you'll find what, and what you should do with it when you're done using it. Here's a theoretical tour of a typical gym.

The Machines

Most gyms are set up sort of like a supermarket—all the equipment that's used for a particular body part is grouped together, just the way all the dairy products are in one aisle. Generally, machines are grouped so that the machines that work larger muscles, like the chest and back, come first, followed by those that work the smaller muscles, like the biceps and triceps. (As we explain later, that's the logical progression for you to follow in your routine.)

Sometimes larger gyms have full lines of more than one brand of machine. If that's the case, you may find all the machines of one line grouped together and the other company's machines in another area. The point is that most gyms have a logical plan that's easy to discern when you know what to look for.

The Free Weights

The dumbbell racks are usually set up in front of a mirror according to weight, with the lighter weights—say, 5- to 50-pound dumbbells—on the top tier and the heavier weights on the bottom tier. (The heaviest dumbbells we've seen in a gym are 150-pounders, which work well as anchors for ocean liners but which you shouldn't even consider trying to lift for some time.)

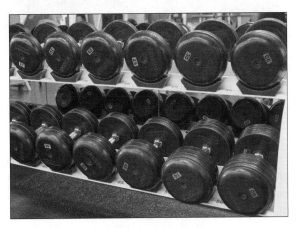

Dumbbell racks in tiers.

Odd-looking treelike objects (vertical racks) also usually are set up adjacent to the location of a barbell. These racks hold metal plates and are (we hope) arranged so the plates that weigh the same amount are grouped together. These plates can be as light as 2½ pounds and as heavy as 45 pounds. Unfortunately, when you're short on time, the 5-pound plate you really want invariably is buried under six 45-pounders—getting that out is a task nearly as arduous as digging out from under a train wreck!

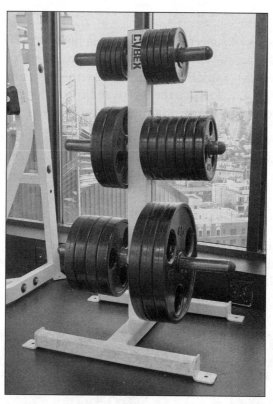

Plates on a tree.

The Bars

The long 45-pound bar used in almost all commercial gyms is called an Olympic bar. These hefty rods of steel are usually found either on the various benches and racks or propped up in a corner. By adding plates to the bar and securing them with collars, you control the amount of weight you lift for any given exercise. Some folks use the bar alone when they bench press; others load as much as 500 pounds onto it. Assuming that you're not working out with someone significantly stronger or weaker than you are (requiring you to remove and replace hundreds of pounds of weight), changing the weight is relatively easy. You just remove the collars, add or subtract weight, and continue on.

For those who aren't ready for a 45-pound bar on a particular exercise, lighter, shorter versions of the Olympic bar are usually available. They are the same diameter and just as compatible with the same set of plates.

Some of the larger and better-equipped gyms have "fixed" barbells in addition to Olympic bars. These bars are already loaded with plates in 5-pound increments and save you the time and trouble of loading and unloading the bar. These usually come in increments ranging from 20 pounds up through 100 pounds. Beyond that, you're back to the bare Olympic bars.

The Pins

Unlike free weights, which are as basic as a hammer and anvil, weight machines have more variables to concern yourself with. In fact, you're bound to encounter machines from lots of companies (Cybex, Nautilus, Bodymaster, Paramount, Maxicam, and more). Luckily, they are more alike than they are different.

Almost all of them are adjusted with pins. Pins are metal rods used to adjust a stack of weights on a particular machine. By placing the pin into a notch on the stack, you set how much weight you'll attempt to lift. Some pins fit straight into the weight stack; others need to be inserted at a certain angle. Other machines require that you push a button before removing or inserting the pin.

Much like socks in a dryer, pins often disappear mysteriously. (Where they go, no one seems to know; because they have virtually no other use, theft is not a viable explanation.) If you're unable to find a pin for the machine you're using, contact a staff member.

One important note: never take a pin from one machine to use with another unless it's of the same model. Because the size and configuration of machines and their weight stacks vary, using the pin from a Universal machine on a Nautilus machine is ill advised. Often the pin pops out, giving you a rude surprise.

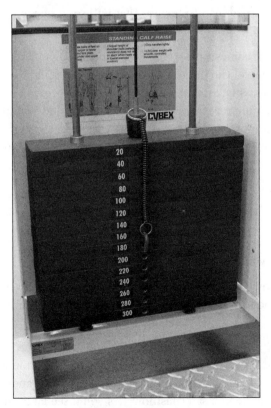

Weight stack using a pin.

Ask First, Lift Later

Some people are comfortable asking questions when they're lost or confused; others (usually men!) remain silent, even if it means they must wander aimlessly for hours. Much to our surprise, we consistently see people working out who clearly are clueless when it comes to the nuances of a particular machine. "Nuances, my ear," you say. "This is a gym, not an art gallery!" Well, okay, let's just say that nearly every piece of equipment can be adjusted in a variety of ways. For example, many benches can be set to a different angle, certain machines can be adjusted to your specifications, and some bars are better suited for certain exercises than others. It can be confusing until you learn which end is up.

Just as you wouldn't wander aimlessly around your workplace during the first week on the job, you shouldn't work out at the gym trying to figure out each piece of equipment for yourself. It seems rather obvious, but when in doubt, ask someone who clearly knows what's what—preferably a staff member.

One way to avoid confusion when you first start out is to take advantage of new member orientations. During these orientations, a staff member takes you through each workout apparatus and shows you how to adjust it to your level of skill and your specific physique. In addition, many gyms offer a workout log, with each setting and adjustment recorded on a card, to help guide you during future visits. You can consider this a road map to terrain that will soon become as familiar to you as your own backyard.

Similarly, don't be shy when it comes time to ask someone to be your spotter. (A spotter is someone who stands by to help you control the weight, in case you reach failure in the middle of a repetition.) This ensures that you don't get stuck under a weight that's too heavy for you to remove. A good spotter can help you squeeze out an extra repetition or two and aid you in getting the most out of each exercise, but the most important role a spotter plays is to ensure safety. One of the advantages of machines over free weights is that machines are generally safer and, unless you want someone to help you squeeze out a few extra repetitions, don't require a spotter for the sake of safety.

When do you use a spotter?

- If you're doing an exercise that you can't walk away from if you "fail" in the middle of a rep.

- If you want to get a little extra out of your workout. Your spotter can help you do a few assisted reps so that you don't have to quit as soon as you're out of gas.

- If you want to see how many repetitions you can get at a certain weight. Say, for example, that you want to bench-press 135 pounds 12 times but aren't confident that you can do more than 10.

Finally, if a spotter isn't available, wait until a staff member or trusted fellow exerciser near you is available. In the meantime, don't just sit around; consider whether another exercise can do the trick by working the same muscle in a safer fashion. (As you'll see later, just about every free weight exercise has a machine equivalent.)

The Collars

Collars are metal clips that you put on the barbell to keep the plates from falling off the bar and onto a part of the human anatomy. They also ensure that you don't break the plates, the floor, or anything else if they come flying off the bar due to recklessness and gravity.

Collars come in several types—some are squeezed on, others are clamped—but they all serve the same purpose. It doesn't really matter what type of collar you use, as long as you use something. At some point in your gym career, you're likely to see some thick-chested guy lifting serious weight on the bench press without collars to secure the weight. With each bounce of the bar on his chest (a big no-no), the plates drift farther toward the end of the barbell. This is a disaster in the making—especially if one of these behemoths is squatting 500 pounds. If one of the plates comes sliding off, it would be next to impossible to maintain balance. With that much weight on the shoulders, a serious injury to the lifter is inevitable, and anyone in the way of the plates is in trouble, too. (For whatever it's worth, we've rarely seen a woman shun collars on an exercise where it was necessary. If we have to shame the guys into proper collar use, so be it.)

In later chapters, we introduce you to some more advanced equipment, but for now, it's important to be familiar with the basics of machines and free weights.

Miss Manners Says …

As a whole, human beings are a sensitive lot. The lack of civility in any locale—while driving in rush-hour traffic, waiting in line at the post office, or working at your desk—is often quite upsetting. The gym is no exception. We can't stress enough the importance of functioning politely and courteously in a setting where you're likely to see many of the same faces day after day. Of course, the basic manners of normal society apply in the gym: no belching, passing gas, or other discourteous behavior is acceptable. However, you should know a few particular items of gym protocol to make everyone's life under the fitness roof more enjoyable—including your own.

Deidre and Joe know a hulking chap who was offended by a woman who refused to let him "work in" with her. (We discuss "working in" in a moment.) Here's a man who has worked out faithfully for more than 20 years, a man who has a shaved head and more muscles than most Rodin sculptures—in short, an intimidating figure—and yet her rude dismissal left him as wounded as a little boy excluded from a game of pickup basketball. "I can't believe that," he muttered over and over as he got madder and madder. Civility is important—on the road, in the workplace, and in the gym.

We also know a man who often bellows so loud in the gym on his last few repetitions that one fears for anyone with a weak heart. Lest you think we're exaggerating, the roar is an obnoxious combination of a martial arts expert breaking bricks and an elephant orgy. Simply put, it's noise pollution.

Lightening the Load

Without question, one of the most common mistakes people make in the gym is leaving "their" weights on the bar when they're finished using them. Even if you're using only a pair of 10-pound weights, it's rude to leave them.

Actually, the people irked the most by this lack of gym courtesy are the staff members who work there. (Jonathan, who worked in gyms for 15 years, often did more lifting while cleaning up after gym members than during his own workouts.) People who regularly abuse their bit of gym protocol say that they're "too busy" or that they "plan to use the bar later" in their workout. Sorry. Imagine a slender woman (who is probably just as busy) spending time hoisting 45-pound plates off a bar you just used. Be fair, and put back what you put on.

May I?

"Working in" with another person using the same piece of equipment you desire is one of the subtle practices in the gym that you need to learn to feel at home. Let's say that you want to do three sets of biceps curls on the biceps machine. If no one is waiting to use it, it's just fine to sit down and wait until you're ready to lift for your next set. However, if someone is waiting to use the machine, it's common courtesy to ask him if he'd like to "work in" with you. (That is, if he doesn't ask you first.) Unless you were just about to start your next set, proper gym etiquette dictates that you get off the equipment and allow the polite interloper to do a set. When he's finished a set, it's your turn. It can seem like an inconvenience, but working in with someone ensures that you don't dawdle between sets, which means you're likely to get a better workout. In the spirit of cooperation, it's a good idea to replace the pin at the weight the other person was using. Ditto on the seat height if you moved it.

Wiping It Clean

Here's another bit of obvious advice that's often ignored: wipe your sweat off the piece of equipment you've just used. Surprisingly, it's a practice that's frequently ignored. It's standard practice to work out with a small towel, bandana, or piece of paper towel. Some people place the towel between them and the seat or bench they're up against. Some just wipe it down after they're done. As long as the sweat is gone, either way is fine.

The "sweating-on-the-equipment" phenomenon can be a touchy one, and some people clearly go overboard, audibly sighing as they wipe the very machine you've just thoroughly toweled off. Our experience is to let them do the extra housework and hope they get to a therapist who can help them deal with their intense reaction to the thought of someone else's perspiration.

Keep It Clean

Gyms have their own unique aroma. People sweat when they lift weights; run on treadmills; ride stationary bikes; and toil away on stair climbers, VersaClimbers, and rowing and cross-country ski machines. Just writing about it is enough to make one break into a cold sweat. All this sweat can turn a poorly maintained gym into a very pungent environment. Most gyms, however, wash their machines with aromatic cleaning fluid and both vacuum and scour the locker rooms.

Sweating is basic to a gym, but don't push your luck by wearing workout gear you've worn three days in a row. This is a good way to earn nicknames like "The Stinky Guy." And it's not advisable if you're planning to run for political office. In fact, wearing foul clothes will …

- Make it difficult to build friendships—at least friends with a sense of smell.
- Make finding a spotter tougher than finding Godot.
- Make you the topic of gym gossip.
- Make it highly unlikely that someone will work in with you.

Of course, as we just said, this is a gym, not an opera house. The idea is to go there and sweat. And although no one expects you to leave smelling like a daisy, it's important that you and your clothing at least start out nose friendly. If you haven't showered in 45 hours, avoid sleeveless shirts and please don't use the gym as the place to find out if your new deodorant's 48-hour guarantee really works.

The Least You Need to Know

- If you've been sick or injured or haven't exercised in years, get a physical before embarking on a new exercise regimen.
- Haven't been sick in years? Take the PAR-Q before you hit the gym.
- After you've received medical clearance, ailments such as diabetes and asthma shouldn't hold you back.
- Fortify your brittle bones, tricky knee, and bad back with a well-designed strength-training regimen.
- Proper technique and attention to detail ensure your safety in the gym.
- How do you learn all the nuances of all those machines? Ask. Learning what goes where is easier than you might think.
- Working in. Wiping off. Smelling clean. It's downright civilized.

Revving the Engine

In This Chapter

- Beginning a stretching program
- Stretching easy and breathing hard
- Learning how to stretch different muscles

Steve Ilg, a highly sought-after professional trainer and author of *The Winter Athlete* (Johnson Books, 1999), has been a nationally sponsored multisport athlete who has excelled in technical rock and ice climbing, Nordic skiing, cycling, and snowshoeing. He is also a yoga teacher and Joe Glickman's coach. Often when he's asked about the best way to stay flexible, he replies, "Renounce your furniture. Learn the Asian squat and make use of it." It might sound absurd or amusing, but it makes sense. If you toss your chairs and tables, reduce the amount of desktop work you do, and eat your meals seated cross-legged on the floor, your lower back and hips will be far better off than in the compressed lifestyle to which most of us are accustomed.

Although getting rid of your furniture might be good for your overall flexibility, it's likely to make your family and friends think that either you've had a momentous religious experience or you're absconding with company funds and heading to Mexico. Assuming that you keep your dining room set and La-Z-Boy lounger, you'll be well served to do the next best thing: embark on a regular stretching program.

"But I hate to stretch," you say. Sure, stretching can be tedious. Plus, it hurts—at least, when you first do it. And wine tastes like cough medicine the first dozen times you try it. However, the more you do it, the more limber your body becomes. Eventually, you'll get so accustomed to and even fond of that self-lubricated sensation that you'll crave it like a Frenchman does a fine Bordeaux.

If you're like the three of us—highly motivated fitness addicts who lead busy lives—here's the way you probably think: *Time is precious—gotta get in and out of the gym as soon as possible.* However, let us assure you (and we're speaking from experience here) that if you don't stretch and continue to work out, your body will rebel. Again, to quote Mr. Ilg, "More than a fitness quality that allows you to gain something, kinesthetic training enables you to release something that is already within." To borrow terminology from the martial arts: lifting weights is *hard* training; stretching is *soft*. Do both, and you're armed and dangerous.

It might sound dramatic, but almost more than anything else we tell you in this book, warming up and stretching are crucial if you're to stay healthy and achieve your fitness goals. Joe, who spends a lot of time crunching his 6-foot, 4-inch frame into a narrow, tippy kayak, suffered from a number of chronic, nagging injuries—the most pernicious being sciatica (a painful condition caused by compressing the sciatic nerve, which is located right behind the back pocket of your pants) in his left leg. Two weeks into his daily stretching routine, the pain virtually disappeared, even though he continued paddling. Ditto for the achy feeling he experienced each morning in his lower back.

This chapter guides you through the basics of warming up and stretching—the two most neglected aspects of the fitness game.

Warming Up: How Long Do I Stay on This Thing?

Years ago, runners and cyclists were taught to head out the door and hit the pavement at full stride—or, at least, to reach peak speed as fast as possible. (Hence the "no pain, no gain" theory.) This might work if you're a Marine in boot camp, but it's a great way to tweak cold muscles and put yourself on the disabled list faster than you can say "illiotibial band syndrome." (ITBS is a common running injury that affects the tissue that runs from the hip to the knee, and it's often alleviated by stretching.) In time, virtually all athletes learned the virtue of a proper warm-up. You should, too.

Warming up is the perfect catchall phrase for what you should do right after you enter the gym and change into your workout gear. Pick your favorite piece of aerobic equipment and ease into an easy-to-maintain rhythm for approximately 10 minutes (although 5 minutes is better than nothing).

Here are our favorite machines to warm up on:

- **The Concept II rowing machine.** This machine works your whole body.

- **A treadmill.** Put it on an easy setting and up a slight (2–3 percent grade), and tread lightly.

- **An elliptical trainer.** This is a great, nonimpact way to get the blood flowing. Machines that use your arms as well as your legs are even better for a warm-up.

How fast should you go? That depends on how fit you are. In other words, if you're breathing heavily, you're going too fast. If your pulse is the same as it is while you're reading this book (unless you're reading it as you ride the exercise bike), you're going too slow. Your aim is to raise your body temperature and increase the blood flow to your muscles and joints. Just as you begin to sweat, it's time to move on to the next crucial stage of working out: stretching.

Hey, Stretch!

When you've finished warming up, head to the stretching area. Typically, this is a small, quiet room littered with mats. You'll know you're in the right place when you hear the loud "whoosh" of people exhaling.

Again, we can't overstress the importance of stretching to both the quality of your workout and the quality of your life. Here's where you stretch each major muscle group. If the mere thought fills you with dread, it's all the more reason to suck it up and face your tight hamstrings.

Kids are naturally as loose as Gumby, but age and our sedentary lifestyles shorten our muscles. Think about it: you sit for hours each day and lie virtually motionless in bed for eight or so hours at a time. Riding a bike, running, and clicking the keyboard of a computer shorten your muscles over the course of a lifetime. Without stretching, the natural length of a muscle changes. This can lead to weakness and muscle imbalances, which, in turn, can lead to structural changes as you get older. Just thinking about it conjures up images of the Hunchback of Notre Dame.

The way to counteract this process is to stretch. Simply put, stretching maintains the flexibility that's compromised as we age. Flexibility is important in both everyday activities (like turning your head before you make a left turn onto the highway, and bending and picking up your 2-year-old child) and athletic endeavors (such as fielding a ground ball and shushing down the ski slopes without pulling a muscle).

In her work as a physical therapist, Deidre sees countless injuries that are directly related to decreased flexibility. Not surprisingly, virtually every one of these injured people complained about lower-back pain. Care to guess how flexible they were? If you said "Not very," you win a complimentary tube of Ben Gay. After they adopted a comprehensive stretching routine, their symptoms usually disappeared.

Now, while Deidre told her patients to stretch like there was no tomorrow, she lifted weights each day and diligently skipped stretching herself. The result? During her powerlifting career, she suffered from chronic lower-back pain. When she was evaluated, she was told that the flexibility of her lower-back musculature was that of a 75-year-old driving instructor. When she began to stretch on a regular basis, this nagging injury receded into the background.

FLEX FACTS

One of the best indicators of back pain and/or potential injury is the sit-and-reach test, in which a subject sits on the floor with straight legs and bends forward at the waist toward his or her toes. If your fingertips can't reach your toes, it's a sure sign that you need to work on your hamstring and lower-back flexibility. If you can't reach your knees, get to a yoga class.

Easy Does It

One of the reasons motivated types like Jonathan and Joe postponed stretching for so long is that they viewed it as a cardio- or strength-training session. They saw it as a contest they waged with themselves (a particularly male condition known as *machismo*). This ability to try less hard is particularly irksome for these achievement types because they are so conditioned to believe that harder is better.

Here's where the train hard/train soft mind-set must come in. The key words when it comes to flexibility training are *gradual* and *easy!* And as we discuss in a moment, the operative phrase is *belly breath.* Stretching consists of several fluid, graceful movements that you do in concert with focused breathing. When you stretch correctly, you should experience mild discomfort in one or more muscle groups, but not pain. If you have pain, you won't get gain.

Why? Inside your muscles are defense mechanisms called muscle spindles. These muscle spindles are quite sensitive to stretching. If your muscle stretches too far too fast, the muscle spindles pull back to shorten the muscle and prevent muscle or tendon damage. This self-protective mechanism makes it so important to stretch correctly. Try too hard, and you may actually end up with less flexibility rather than more.

To Do and Not to Do

Although most of us did it in high school gym class, bouncing while you stretch has gone the way of the beehive hairdo. It might have seemed like a good idea at the time, but we know much better these days.

If you bounce while stretching, you're likely to engage those defensive mechanisms or, worse yet, override them and pull a muscle. To state the obvious, don't bounce—it won't help your flexibility.

Consider the three most important points to remember about basic stretching:

1. Stretch to the point that you feel a gentle tension in the muscle. That sounds like a contradiction in terms, but it's really another way of saying that you should ease into a mild state of discomfort, well short of pain.

2. Hold the stretch for 20 to 30 seconds.

3. As you hold the stretch, breathe deeply, stretching just a little farther with each exhalation.

It seems somewhat silly to mention, but it's crucial to remember to breathe while you stretch. Breathing helps deliver fresh blood to your muscles. Get into the habit of practicing this deep-belly breathing because it will help you immensely when you lift weights. However, it's common practice to hold your breath as you move deeper into a stretch. Be mindful of this—it's a sign that you're pushing too hard or are resistant to the task at hand—and return to your breath. Not only will this help you relax, but it will allow you to stretch a little farther with each exhalation.

Deep breathing is not something we do naturally at rest. In fact, most of us breathe shallowly from the chest and don't use our diaphragm. Try this now: place one hand on your abdomen and one hand on your chest. Take a deep breath through your nose, and fill your abdomen with air (you should feel your hand rise with your abdomen). Complete the breath by filling your chest with air (you should feel your hand rise with your chest). Now exhale through your mouth, expelling air from your abdomen first and then from your chest. Repeat this slowly five times. You may feel a little dizzy or light-headed, but that's normal because you're not used to such oxygenated air.

Of course, you're not going to place your hand on your abdomen or your chest while you stretch or lift weights. (It's challenging enough to lift with two hands, let alone one.) Instead, practice inhaling deeply through your nose and forcefully out through your mouth. When you realize the positive effect this has on your stretching (not to mention your sense of well-being), it will be a standard part of your workout.

Now that we've convinced you of the importance of getting (and staying) limber, let's take a look at some of our favorite stretches. Starting a routine is a little like working your way into a great book. The first 50 pages may seem laborious, but when you get into it, you'll be hard pressed to put it down. Do the following for two weeks. You'll be surprised by how grateful your stiff body feels.

Torso Stretch

Improving and maintaining a flexible trunk (torso) is extremely important, for obvious reasons. If you've ever seen an elderly person (or someone with a back injury) bend down to pick up a piece of paper, you'll know what we mean. If your torso becomes stiff, simple tasks such as turning and reaching are compromised. In fact, you often hear of people who say they "threw out" their backs lifting a pot of water. In fact, that was merely the straw that broke the camel's back.

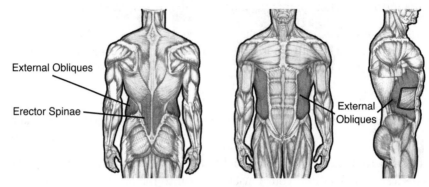

External Obliques

Erector Spinae

External Obliques

Torso stretch: muscles used.

SPOT ME

For people who have scoliosis (sideways curvature of the spine), the torso stretch is a good stretch for the opposite side of the curvature. For example, for a left-sided scoliosis, you should stretch the right side.

Here's what you need to do to stretch your torso:

1. Stand with your feet shoulder width apart and your toes pointed straight ahead.

2. Keep your knees bent slightly.

3. Place one hand on your hip for support while you extend your other arm up and over your head toward the ceiling.

4. Now slowly bend at your waist to the side where your hand rests on your hip.

5. Move slowly and gracefully, and continue to breathe.

6. Hold the stretch for 20 to 30 seconds.

7. Repeat on the other side.

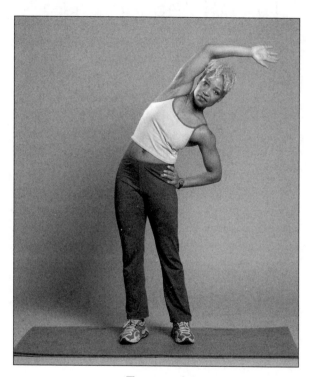

Torso stretch.

Pec Stretch

This is a good stretch to do at any time, especially if you're at a desk and find yourself slumping.

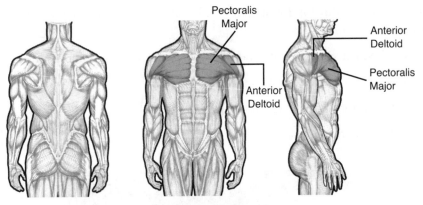

Pec stretch: muscles used.

SPOT ME

The pec stretch is a great stretch for people who suffer from asthma. Asthmatics tend to take on a forward chest posture, probably from difficulty breathing. This stretch opens up the chest muscles, freeing the muscles used for breathing.

Here's what you need to do to stretch your pectoral muscles, the muscles of your chest that pull your arms forward:

1. Stand or sit on a bench, and interlace your fingers behind your back.

2. Lift your arms behind you until you feel a stretch in your arms, shoulders, and chest.

3. Keep your chest out and your chin in.

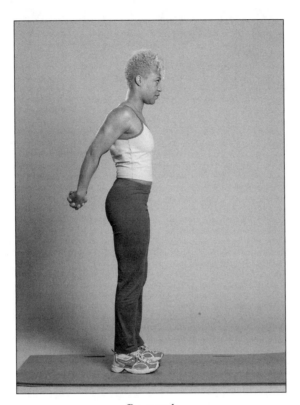

Pec stretch.

Spinal Twist

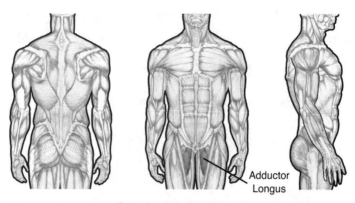

Adductor
Longus

Spinal twist: muscles used.

The spinal twist is great for limbering the muscles that align your spinal column. It also stretches the buttocks and hips. Here's how to do it:

1. Sit with your left leg straight on the floor.

2. Place your right foot flat on the floor over your outstretched left leg, and rest it to the outside of your left knee.

3. Place your left elbow on the outside of your upper right thigh, just above your knee.

4. With your right hand resting behind you, slowly turn your head and look over your right shoulder. At the same time, rotate your upper body toward your right hand and arm.

5. During the stretch, use your left elbow to keep your right leg stationary, with controlled pressure to the inside. As you turn your upper body, think of turning your hips in the same direction without lifting your hips off the floor. You should feel a stretch in your lower back and the side of your hip.

6. Hold for 20 to 30 seconds.

7. Breathe deeply. Repeat on the opposite side.

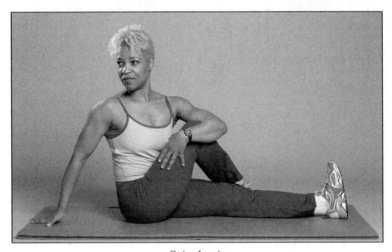

Spinal twist.

Groin Stretch

Tight groin muscles are a common source of strains in sports with sudden stops, starts, and turns. The groin is defined as the depression between the thigh and the trunk, and consists primarily of tendons from your *adductor* muscles.

DEFINITION

The **adductor** muscles are the muscles that draw your leg in toward your body from an outward position.

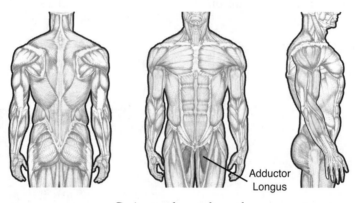

Adductor Longus

Groin stretch: muscles used.

Here's what you need to do to stretch your groin muscles:

1. Sit with your spine straight.

2. Put the soles of your feet together and grab your toes.

3. Bending from your hips, gently pull yourself forward until you feel a good stretch in your groin. Do not make the initial movement for the stretch from your head and shoulders; move from your hips. You may also feel a stretch in your lower back.

4. Hold for 20 to 30 seconds.

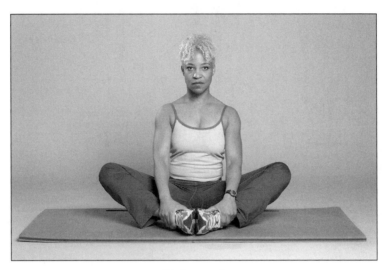

Groin stretch.

Quadriceps Stretch

The quadriceps (or "quads") are a group of four individual muscles—rectus femoris, vastus medialis, vastus lateralis, and vastus intermedius, if you must know—that attract so much attention when you walk around in shorts. They work together to straighten the knee. The rectus femoris is the only muscle of the four that crosses the hip. Your quads are the workhorses in activities such as running, stair climbing, squatting, and lunging.

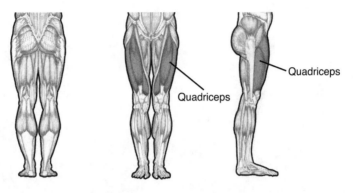

Quadriceps stretch: muscles used.

To stretch these large muscles, do the following:

1. Stand near a wall for support.

2. Bend your right knee and hold the top of your right foot with your left hand, gently pulling your heel toward your buttocks. Be sure your knee is pointing down toward the floor.

3. Keep your hips and shoulders level.

4. Hold for 20 to 30 seconds.

5. Breathe deeply throughout the stretch and then switch to the other leg.

SPOT ME

The reason you hold your foot with your opposite hand is that the natural angle of the patellofemoral joint is not straight as you bend it; it turns inward with end-range flexion.

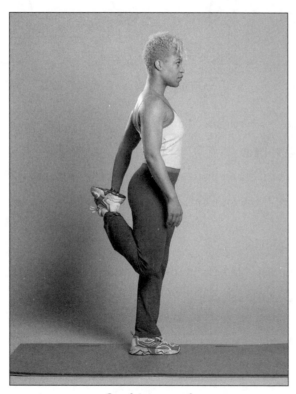

Quadriceps stretch.

Hamstring Stretch

The hamstrings are three individual muscles that oppose the quads—the biceps femoris, semitendinosus, and semimembranosus, for those of you keeping score at home. They work as a group to bend the knee and straighten the hip. Tight hamstrings, a condition so common that it sounds like the official name, can often contribute to low-back pain. Keep them loose, and you'll feel like a new person.

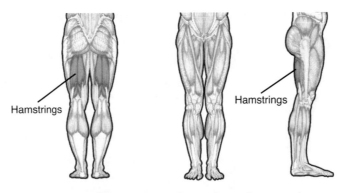

Hamstring stretch: muscles used.

Here's what you need to do to stretch your hamstrings:

1. Sit and straighten your right leg.

2. Place the sole of your left foot against the inside of your right thigh.

3. Slowly bend forward from your hips toward the foot of your outstretched leg until you feel a gentle stretch.

4. Hold for 20 to 30 seconds.

5. When the initial discomfort has diminished, bend forward a bit more.

6. Hold for another 20 to 30 seconds.

Again, when the stretch becomes more comfortable, lean forward for the last time for another 20 to 30 seconds. Repeat this three-part move on your other leg. Remember to relax and focus on your breathing.

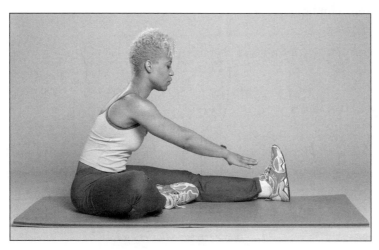

Hamstring stretch.

Hip Flexor Stretch

Next we have the hip flexor, as it is called in lay terms; to medical types, it refers to the iliopsoas muscle, which flexes the hip. The hip flexors are instrumental in running, especially sprinting, as well as cycling and stair climbing.

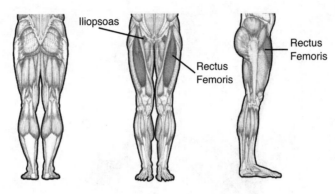

Hip flexor stretch: muscles used.

Here's how you work your hip flexors:

1. Kneel on both knees.

2. Extend one leg forward so that the knee of your forward leg forms a right angle directly over your ankle.

3. Gently lower the front of your hip so that your back leg lies on the ground like an L.

4. Hold for 20 to 30 seconds.

5. Switch legs and work your other hip.

Be careful of this stretch if you have knee problems. Here's a fine alternative to that stretch:

1. Stand facing a support high enough that your hip and knee form a 90° angle.

2. Bend your left knee and place your left foot on the support.

3. Keep your grounded foot pointed straight ahead.

4. Keeping your back straight, lean your hips forward until the heel of your standing foot lifts slightly from the floor.

5. You should feel a slight stretch in the front of your right hip. Hold for 20 to 30 seconds.

6. Repeat on your other leg.

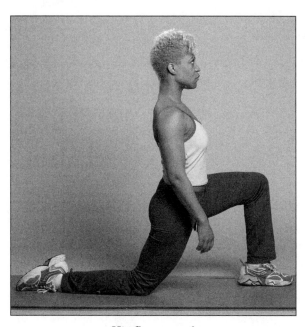

Hip flexor stretch.

Calf Stretch

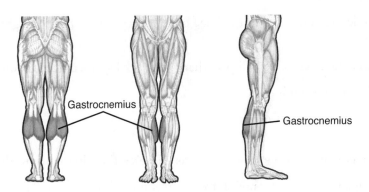

Gastrocnemius stretch: muscles used.

To stretch your gastrocnemius (the calf, to you and me), do the following:

1. Stand on a solid support and lean forward against a wall.

2. Place one bent leg forward and extend the other leg, with a straight knee, behind.

3. Slowly move your hips forward, keeping your lower back flat.

4. Be sure to keep the heel of your straight leg on the ground, with your toes pointed straight ahead.

5. Hold for 20 to 30 seconds.

6. Don't bounce, be sure you breathe, and repeat on the other side.

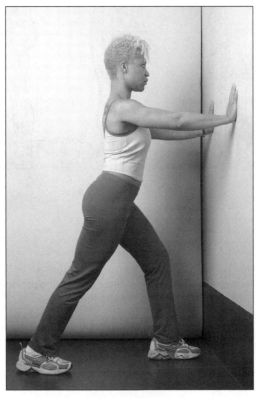

Gastrocnemius stretch.

WEIGHT A MINUTE

For any stretch in which you have to bend your knee, be absolutely certain that your knee doesn't "over-shoot" your toe. The knee should never be farther forward than your toes; otherwise, there's too much stress on your knee.

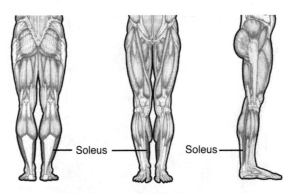

Soleus stretch: muscles used.

SPOT ME

Tight hamstrings and tight calves (also called the gastrocnemius) can be the source of a knee condition called *patellofemoral syndrome*. Symptoms can include pain during prolonged sitting and walking down stairs. Getting these muscles flexible can help alleviate this problem.

Here's a wrinkle to the gastrocnemius stretch to work the deeper calf muscle as well as the Achilles tendon:

1. Assume the position we just described for the gastrocnemius stretch, but lower your hips as you slightly bend your back knee and bring it forward just a touch.

2. Be sure to keep your back flat.

3. Try to keep the heel of your back foot down.

4. Hold for 20 to 30 seconds.

5. Switch legs and stretch the other side.

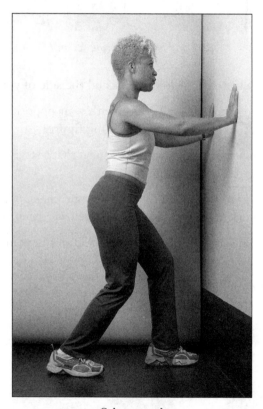

Soleus stretch.

Back and Hip Stretch

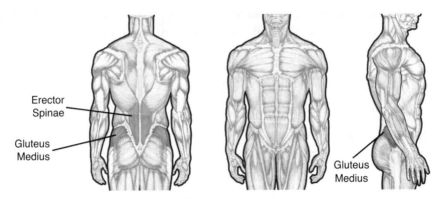

Erector
Spinae

Gluteus
Medius

Gluteus
Medius

Back and hip stretch: muscles used.

Here's what you need to do to stretch your lower back and the side of your hip:

1. Lie on your back, bend one knee at 90°, and, with your opposite hand, pull that bent leg up and over your other leg, as shown in the following figure.

2. Turn your head to look toward the hand of the arm that's straight out, palm down (your head should be resting on the floor, not held up).

3. Placing the other hand on your thigh (just above your knee), pull your bent leg toward the floor until you feel the right stretch feeling in your lower back and side of hip.

4. Keep your feet and ankles relaxed, and be sure the backs of your shoulders are flat on the floor.

5. Hold for 20 to 30 seconds, and repeat on the other side.

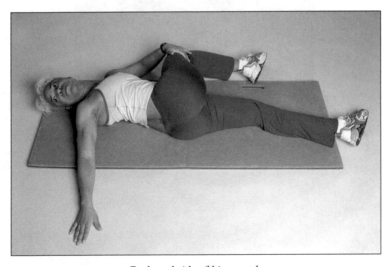

Back and side of hip stretch.

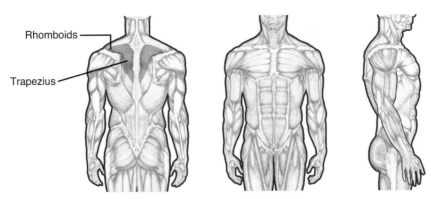

Rhomboids

Trapezius

Middle back stretch: muscles used.

Here's what you need to do to stretch your middle back:

1. Stand and interlace your fingers in front of you at shoulder height.

2. Turn your palms outward as you extend your arms forward, as if pushing something away from you.

3. You should feel a stretch in your shoulders, the middle of your upper back, and your arms, hands, fingers, and wrists.

4. Hold for 20 to 30 seconds, and repeat twice.

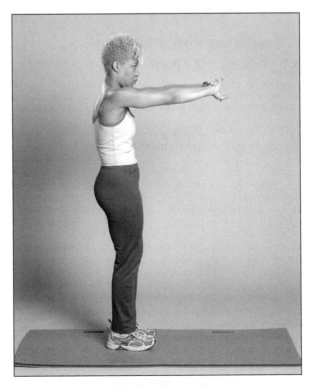

Middle back stretch.

Advanced Techniques

Static stretching is the most proven and safe method of increasing flexibility, but you may come across other techniques in the gym. As we mentioned earlier, bouncing, or ballistic stretching, can be unsafe and ineffective, so we never advocate it. But other, more advanced stretching methods that can further your quest for flexibility.

Dynamic stretching is a method that takes the muscle through a range of motion, but not to the point at which your defense mechanisms fire. It's an increasingly popular way to stretch, and many physiologists find it more effective than static stretching before exercise.

In active isolated stretching, a technique developed by Jim and Phil Wharton, the exerciser moves through a full range of motion by contracting the opposing muscle while stretching. The stretch is held for only a few seconds and then is repeated.

Proprioceptive neuromuscular facilitation is a technique more commonly used in therapeutic settings, but it has gained popularity among some personal trainers as well. It temporarily fools your defense mechanisms as you strongly contract the muscle you plan to stretch immediately before you do so.

Each of these techniques is a viable way to stretch but should be treated with respect. A class or session with a trainer who is versed in these techniques is advisable before trying them.

The Least You Need to Know

- Age and a sedentary lifestyle make stretching a necessity.
- Stretch to the point at which you feel a gentle tension in the muscle.
- Hold your stretches for at least 20 seconds.
- As you hold the stretch, breathe deeply, stretching just a little farther with each exhalation.
- Whether you're hustling after a bus or trying out for the Bolshoi Ballet, you'll feel and perform far better if you're limber from the waist down.

The Workout

It's funny how many people who start lifting have little or no idea what muscles they're working. "I want to work these things," they say, pointing to their deltoids. In Part 2, you'll find a thorough list of weightlifting exercises for your entire body. Each exercise is accompanied by photos and a detailed explanation of what to do. Why is it important to hold your elbows here or your knees there? And while we generally stick with the basics, we'll also introduce you to some more advanced techniques and equipment that can spice up your workouts, as well as ways to stay in shape even if you can't make it to the gym. Part 2, which tells you how and why, is your own personal trainer guiding you in print.

Gluteus What?

In This Chapter

- Learning the lingo
- Standing, bending, and sitting at your own risk
- Breathing big
- Remembering technique, technique, technique

Each sport, club, fraternity, and family (and any other subset of society-at-large) seemingly has its own lingo, its own code words that the initiated use as shorthand. Cyclists "hammer," "jam," or "bonk"; street hoop junkies "slam," "dish," and do battle in "the paint." The gym, of course, has its own jargon. Words such as *pecs*, *quads*, and *lats* are tossed around like 5-pound barbells. These code words may sound like snippets of conversation between two narcotics cops, but they're actually abbreviated versions of the technical names for various body parts.

When Joe was a child, his uncle gave him an anatomy book he'd used during medical school. Each page revealed another complete system: circulatory, nervous, muscular, and so on. As a child, pondering how these separate systems functioned as one filled him with wonder. Even as a busy adult, when you pause to consider the human body, only the most jaded mortician wouldn't be awed by the complexity of this amazing machine. Because you're going to be spending a fair bit of time working your muscles, we think it's important to be able to visualize what's going on beneath your epidermis. In fact, the better you understand how your muscles work, the easier it is to appreciate what we're talking about when it comes to particular exercises. In addition, gaining an appreciation for human anatomy might motivate you to maintain solid technique and avoid injuring yourself.

In this chapter, we provide you with charts so you can familiarize yourself with the roughly 600 muscles that comprise your body, the very muscles you'll become intimately involved with in the near future.

Know What and Where It Is

Here's a partial list of common code words you'll hear at the gym:

- **Pecs (pectoralis major).** This is the body part Fabio made famous. In ancient Greece, soldiers were chided, "What do you want, a medal or pecs to pin it on?" The pecs are the muscles of your chest and move the upper arm down and across the body.

- **Lats (latissimus dorsi).** Check out a world-class swimmer or kayaker from behind, and you'll see the sweeping expanse of muscle from the armpit to just above the waist that resembles a highly agitated cobra. The lats pull the upper arm back and down.

- **Quads (quadriceps).** Back in his racing days, from the waist up, Jonathan looked like a fairly normal athletic human being. (Of course, looks can be deceiving.) However, from the waist down, he looked a bit like two loaves of bread with too much yeast. Why? As a cyclist who averaged 5,000 miles a year, his quads were his biggest allies. The quads' main function is straightening the knee.

- **Hams or hammies (hamstrings).** Look at any Olympic sprinter's muscular legs for an example of what hamstrings can look like. Hamstrings, which are made up of three separate muscles that run from just beneath the backside to the back of the knee, are responsible for bending the knee—and they're as inflated as a side of beef in most of these guys. In fact, all superior sprinters and NFL running backs, and other people who regularly need a burst of speed, have these sweeping, sculpted strands of muscle.

- **Bi's (biceps).** Large biceps (guns), the muscle that bunches up into a ball between your elbow and shoulder, are the classic symbol of masculine strength. What do Madonna, Mr. Olympia, and Mr. Clean have in common? Big biceps! Without them, the tattoo business would be in dire straits. The biceps are to the arms what the hamstrings are to the legs—they bend your elbow.

- **Tri's (triceps).** The opposing muscle to the more famous biceps, triceps push while the biceps pull. This lopsided triangle of muscle on the posterior side of your upper arm is most visible when you do a push-up. The job of the triceps is to straighten your elbow.

- **Traps (trapezius).** If you've ever seen Mike Tyson sans shirt, you've likely noticed these two Brahma bull–like lumps that sprout from under his ears and connect to the tops of his shoulders. These pronounced loaves of muscle help shrug your shoulders and pull your shoulder blades together.

- **Delts (deltoids).** Atlas shrugged them, and we call them delts. It's the shoulder muscle, a large triangle-shaped muscle that covers the joint and serves to raise the arm laterally.

FLEX FACTS

The word *deltoid* is derived from the Greek word *delta*, which means "triangle." Take a look at a well-developed pair of delts, and you'll see why.

- **Abs (rectus abdominis).** Also known as the tummy, gut, and stomach—which actually is a misnomer—your abdominals run from the lower rim of the rib cage to the pelvis. Your stomach is the organ that digests your food. Well-developed "six-pack" abs à la Bruce Lee not only look great, but also increase your athletic potency tenfold.

- **Glutes (gluteus maximus).** *Buttocks, tush, backside, derriere,* and many more are synonyms for this old trusted friend. Once developed, these oft-neglected muscles provide lots of *oomph* for forward propulsion.

Here's a nuance of gym vernacular you should know about. Typically, when someone is asked what body parts he's working on a particular day, the answer is something like "chest and back, shoulders and arms," and so on. Rarely will you hear someone say, "I'm working my pecs and delts." However, when lifters refer to a particular body part, they often use the abbreviated Latin names we've just mentioned. For example, you might hear, "Wow, your lats are huge," or "Your abs are ripped," or "Your quads look like a chicken that needs a tan." (Just for the record: the first two are highly complimentary; the latter is a solid insult.)

The following is a chart of the muscles of the front (anterior aspect) and back (posterior aspect) of the body.

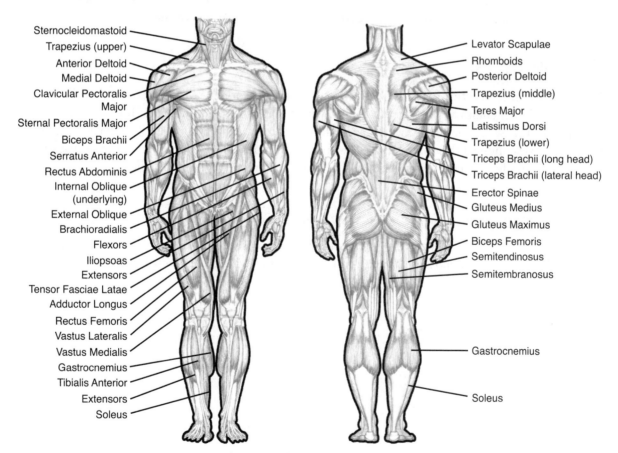

Anterior and posterior muscle chart.

Walking Tall

At first glance, lifting weights is less risky than, say, waterskiing or rock climbing. All you need to do—once you join a gym—is walk in and start lifting. Herein lies the rub. In sports such as waterskiing, the risky elements are obvious: fast boat, hard water, big ouch. Assuming that you don't drop a barbell on your forehead, the risk in weightlifting tends to be cumulative—the proverbial drop in a bucket that one day overflows and stains the carpet.

Take a chap we know at the gym—a short, bearded, muscular guy who trains hard. Regardless of the exercise, he piles on a lot of weight and gives it the old heave-ho. The problem, however, is that he's often twisting and straining and using other body parts to assist him as he reaches failure. Not long ago, he was complaining to Joe about his sore left shoulder. He reduced the amount of weight he used on the bench (a notorious shoulder wanker), but he continued lifting like a man paid by the pound. The moral of the story? Arthroscopic surgery that will keep him out of the gym for six weeks.

As we've now said many times, before you start hoisting weights, you need to be sure that you can able to execute all these exercises with sound form and technique. That means proper posture and attention to your breathing. If you start using shoddy technique, you're likely to build a house of cards. If a strong wind rushes through one day, you'll be reduced to rubble. And remember, it's harder to unlearn bad habits than it is to learn good ones. So learn it here the right way.

Be Erect

Woody Allen once said that his brain was his "second favorite organ." Most men would probably agree, but when it comes to your overall health, your back is the most important body part you have, principally because it's the core to which everything (muscles, nerves, and so on) is attached. As a private-practice physical therapist, Deidre saw many ailing patients who complained about back pain after a particularly strenuous gym workout. The biggest culprit? Lousy technique.

Try this exercise:

1. Stand against a wall so that the back of your head and your buttocks are flush against it.

2. Now take one step forward, tighten your stomach muscles, and keep your buttocks in the same position—almost as though you have a tail tucked between your legs.

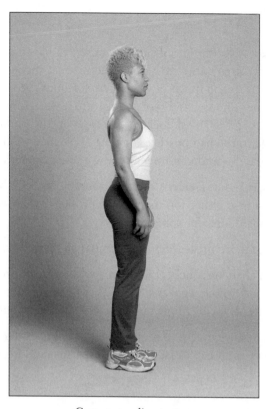

Correct standing posture.

This is the position you should maintain while performing any standing weightlifting exercises. At first you might feel like a Buckingham Palace guard or an English schoolmarm, but once you get used to feeling comfortable like this, you'll be righting a lot of postural wrongs. The bottom line here is that when you're properly aligned, your abdominal muscles help protect your back and decrease excessive *lordosis*, a condition that can be a source of back pain. Bad posture is enough to injure your back, but start stressing your skeleton with weights, and the plot only thickens.

DEFINITION

Lordosis refers to the natural inward curve of the lumbar or lower spine. In some people, especially those with potbellies, the curve is greater than normal and can be the source of back pain.

Sitting Bull

As we have mentioned, an excessive amount of sitting can wreak havoc on your skeletal structure. Let's set the record straight: we aren't anti-sitting—in fact, we sat throughout the writing of this book. However, too many of us sit too much of the time—for hours at work, in front of the television, in the car to Grandmother's house, and more. Most often we are sitting in chairs that are improperly fitted for us, and if you're a desk jockey who talks on the phone a lot, this unnatural position adds another wrinkle to the bad posture formula. Toss in a good dose of stress—"What, the order won't be here till Tuesday?"—and you understand why massage is such a thriving business.

Twenty-five percent of the patients in Deidre's physical therapy practice had back (upper and lower), shoulder, or neck pain from sitting either too much or improperly. How can such a passive activity as sitting cause so many problems? Consider some reasons:

- When we sit, we place more pressure on the lumbar spine than when we stand.

- When we slouch in a chair or couch, the *erector spinae* muscles are overstretched for an extended period of time, which weakens them. Weak muscles tend to spasm because they have to work harder to perform simple tasks such as sitting straight.

- Serious slouchers crane their necks to see what's in front of them. This puts significant pressure on the *cervical spine* and can cause weakness, spasms, and headaches.

DEFINITION

The **erector spinae** muscles run along either side of the spine and are instrumental in good sitting posture. The **cervical spine** is the part of your spine that attaches your head to your body. When someone says, "He's lost his head," he's indirectly talking about the cervical spine. It consists of the first seven vertebrae from the base of your skull (C1) to the largest protrusion you can feel (C7).

Poor posture can also cause shoulder problems. How? Try this: slouch in a chair and raise your arms overhead. Now sit up straight. Notice a difference in your range of motion? Slouching does not allow proper engagement of your rotator cuff muscles, which can weaken them over time and lead to problems such as *impingement syndrome*. Impingement syndrome is a painful shoulder condition that can be caused by several factors, including a weak rotator cuff. As you raise your arm, an arc of pain radiates in your shoulder. Strengthening the weak muscles in the area often resolves the problem.

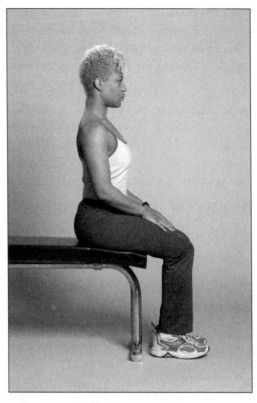

Proper sitting posture.

Bend Right

Let's assume for a moment that, after reading about the various skeletal maladies, you haven't quit your job, sold your furniture, and moved to a yoga ashram to find postural enlightenment. Instead, let's hope that you at least recognize the importance of sitting up correctly and the subsequent importance of stretching. Unfortunately for the poor unsuspecting weightlifter, another danger is lurking in the shadowy recesses of your neighborhood gym: improper bending—probably the number-one cause of lower-back pain. Luckily, it's also the most preventable.

Our backs are built to withstand a tremendous amount of pressure. Our spines, flexible pieces of architectural genius, act as shock absorbers to counteract forces that occur from walking, running, skipping, hopping, driving, sky diving, weightlifting—well, you get the point. However, our backs are not built to withstand the rigors of bending all day long, especially when picking up heavy objects.

If you continually bend the spine of a book in the opposite direction it was meant to go, it eventually weakens and breaks. This is more or less what happens with your spine when you continually use your back incorrectly day after day, year after year. In her private practice, Deidre heard countless times, "I just bent over to pick up my shoe, and my back gave out." Well, that may be the way it seemed, but that's not the way it happened.

"How," you may ask, "should I bend if not from my back?" Ironically, most of us know how to bend correctly because we have ample practice doing so when we have a stiff and sore back. When your back is ailing, you be sure you use your hips and your knees to lower your body to the ground and to raise yourself up again. Your legs have the largest muscle groups in the body for a reason.

All this has considerable practical application to the time you spend in the gym: you have to bend to pick up weights and you have to bend to put them back. To state the obvious: it is very important that you do this correctly.

Try this exercise:

1. Stand against a wall with your feet shoulder width apart, roughly 6 inches from the wall.

2. Begin to slowly slide down the wall while bending your knees.

3. Now step away from the wall and lower yourself into a deep knee bend while keeping your back straight.

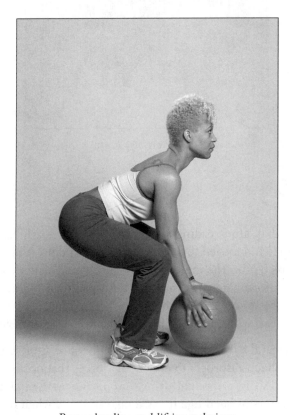

Proper bending and lifting technique.

This is how you should use your back at all times, whether picking up a gum wrapper or lifting a 45-pound barbell.

In and Out

Joe's coach, Steve Ilg, is a big proponent of training an athlete's mind, body, and spirit. Peppered throughout his training schedules are small reminders that pay huge dividends. Here's one to keep in mind whenever you train: "Spine erect, breath full and deep, yet soft."

Breathing properly allows you to merge with the activity at hand. This might sound like a line from *Kung Fu*, but it's one of the most important techniques you can use. Why? The link that connects the body and the mind—a hard-to-describe but easily felt connection—is the breath. Not only will this help you lift more and better, but it is also a key way to alleviate boredom in the gym.

Conversely, breathing shallowly or even holding your breath is like working out while wearing a corset. Done under extreme stress, holding your breath can cause you to black out by cutting off oxygen to your brain. And you increase the chance of having a stroke by aneurysm.

Try this exercise:

1. Inhale deeply through your nose and then exhale through your mouth. Repeat this five times. (If you're not used to breathing from your diaphragm, you may feel a little dizzy.)

2. Sit in a chair with your arms by your side.

3. Inhale through your nose.

4. Raise your arms until they are shoulder level and exhale through your mouth.

5. Lower your arms while inhaling through your nose.

This little exercise is a way to introduce you to how you would be breathing in the gym while performing shoulder raises.

SPOT ME

When you're lifting weights, remember to forcefully exhale in the concentric or power phase. This ensures that you breathe through the most difficult part of the exercise when the tendency is to hold your breath. To help you remember, keep this in mind: exhale on effort.

Up Three, Down Three

Earlier, we referred to the use of momentum as a way to "cheat" when lifting (read: for men eager to lift more than they should). This use of body English (cheating) makes the exercise easier and puts a ton of stress on various joints in your body. It may help you lift more weight, but this jerkiness ensures that you're not giving the specific muscle group proper attention. By using the technique of "up three and down three," you effectively remove momentum from the gym and put it back in Physics 101, where it belongs.

Here's how this simple but effective technique works:

1. Stand with your arms by your side. While bending your elbows, count "one-and-a," "two-and-a," "three-and-a." By the end of "three-and-a," your elbows should be fully bent. Pause for one count at the fully contracted position.

2. Now reverse the process and straighten your elbows. As you do so, count "one-and-a," "two-and-a," "three-and-a." By the end of "three-and-a," your elbows should be straight. (We recommend that you do this silently unless you're a bandleader or a kindergarten teacher.)

This count helps you to move slowly, establish a good rhythm, and ensure that you're depending entirely on the muscles you should be working.

Here's a quick checklist of reminders to take with you on each trip to the gym:

❏ Perform all standing exercises with proper standing posture.

❏ Perform all sitting exercises with proper sitting posture.

❏ Bend from your hips and knees, not your back.

❏ Breathe properly, in through your nose and out through your mouth.

❏ Remember the count—3 seconds on the positive phase of the lift, a 1-second pause, and 3 seconds for the negative.

Improper Technique

Here's a solid bit of irony. After reading the preceding information, you may decide that it's easier to perform exercises improperly, and you're probably right. When you enlist other muscles to assist you, hold your breath, or use momentum to your advantage, the exercise becomes easier, but at a cost—safety and effectiveness.

We want to make this very clear so that you know incorrect technique when you see it. Furthermore, we don't care who's doing it—the huge guy with the bulging biceps or the trainer (yes, the trainer) who is showing an exercise to a novice who doesn't know a dumbbell from a doorbell.

We know a trainer who advises all his clients improperly. In fact, when Deidre hears him tell clients to "throw your back" into a biceps exercise or recommend that they perform leg extensions at break-neck speed, she's tempted to walk over and hand the client her physical therapy business card. The majority of trainers know their stuff, but this is a good reminder that you shouldn't take everything a trainer teaches you as gospel. Don't be afraid to challenge them and have them explain their thought process if you don't understand something. If we question our doctors, we can certainly question health club trainers.

WEIGHT A MINUTE

Using bad form often makes it easy to hoist more weight, but not without a price. The extra weight may make you feel stronger, but it won't really strengthen your muscles. Worse still, bad form makes any exercise more dangerous.

Cheers

Water, water everywhere, but alas, few of us drink enough of the stuff. This is even more applicable for people who work out. The key fact to remember is that by the time you're thirsty, your body is already dehydrated. The trick is to head off that thirsty fiend at the pass and stay topped off in the first place.

If you notice that you're lethargic or sore, or if you experience muscle cramps or irritability after a particularly hard workout, odds are, you're dehydrated. It's recommended that you drink at least 65 ounces (for women) or 80 ounces (for men) of water per day, even if you don't exercise that day. Remember, now that you're increasing your activity level, you must drink more water to maintain proper hydration.

We don't expect you to keep track of how many ounces of water you consume, but an easy way to tell whether you are hydrated is to note the color of your urine. If you're well hydrated, your urine will be virtually colorless (unless you take vitamins). If it's a concentrated yellow and you don't take vitamins, drink up, mate!

You can do as we say or learn the hard way. Take Deidre, the powerlifter who preached the virtues of stretching but who hardly stretched until she was so compromised that she *had* to stretch to get out of bed in the morning. Before training for the New York City Marathon in 1999, she still wasn't convinced that she needed to drink more than a few glasses of water a day—until she completed a 9-mile run that left her wiped out with fatigue and muscle soreness for two days. After several demonstrative vows of "liquid repentance," she heeded this traditional hydro warning and drank the appropriate amount of water for a week before her next long run. Much to her surprise, she felt much better during and after the run. As you no doubt know, there's nothing worse than the zeal of a recent convert!

The Least You Need to Know

- Proper attention to posture—sitting, standing, and bending—is essential.
- Understanding the importance of proper breathing further ensures the mind/body connection.
- Remember that by the time you're thirsty, your body may be on its way to dehydration; the trick is to stay topped off in the first place.

Now What?

In This Chapter

- Understanding physiology fact and fiction
- Determining how long, how much, and how often
- Learning what's in a rep

Strength training is part art, part science, and part luck. The science is how to lift and when. On the physiological front, we know a lot about what happens when you follow specific training guidelines. The art is applying this knowledge to your body. For example, how hard do you lift? Are you able to back off when you're tired and push harder when you're stuck at a plateau? Does your diet complement your fitness goals or sabotage them? A host of other factors also govern one's progress in the game of fitness. The luck part revolves around one word: *genetics*.

In other words, a lot of variables surround a lifting program—some you can obviously control, some you can't. In this chapter, we discuss the various x-factors involved so that you have a better understanding of how you can best progress in the gym. For example, here's a question that continually stumps people: Why do two people who work out together, doing virtually the same routines, progress at different rates? Read on.

That Was Intense!

Having said that, of all the variables in your lifting program, how hard you work—let's call it the intensity factor—is the single most important one you can control. In this chapter, we give you plenty of tips on how to safely increase this intensity factor so that you get better results faster.

Of course, some variables aren't under your control: age, gender, muscle fiber types, and a few other genetically determined variables play a major role in your strength development. We talk about what they are and how you can work *with* them instead of getting frustrated and giving up.

It's Quality, Not Quantity

No real differences exist between the muscle fibers of men and those of women. On a pound-for-pound basis, women are capable of becoming as strong as men. (When Deidre competed as a powerlifter, on a pound-for-pound scale, she routinely outlifted most of the men at the meets.) However, because men tend to be larger and have a greater percentage of lean tissue (lower percentage of body fat), men generally have greater strength potential. Dr. Wayne Westcott put it best: men are stronger than women due to muscle quantity, not muscle quality. There are differences between the sexes, but the methods used to train women need not be any different than those used for men. In fact, the glut of women's exercise programs arises more from a marketing angle than from genuine need.

How Long?

Consider this scenario: identical twins Tim and Tom are seated on opposite sides of a seesaw. If Tim sits all the way at the end while Tom sits 3 feet from the end, Tom will be airborne despite the fact they are exactly the same size. It's an issue of simple physics.

Now picture two workout partners who have been training together for one year. Let's say they're doing biceps curls. If both lifters are using the same weight and lifting with the same intensity, one may outlift the other by a substantial margin. Why? Again, it's physics, because the lifter with the shorter arms has much less work to do. Clearly, there's no reason for the longer-armed lifter to alter his training program—and reducing your arm length is far too drastic a course to follow—but it explains why the shorter-armed chap is progressing at a faster rate.

Now here's one you've probably not spent a lot of time pondering: tendon length. Remember that tendons attach muscle to bone. Let's consider the biceps curl again to show how tendon length can affect strength. The biceps muscle runs from the shoulder to a point just below the elbow. Sparing you the physiological details, you might be interested to know that if your tendon attaches farther from the elbow, it's analogous to being at the far end of the seesaw. Similarly, an attachment closer to the joint is analogous to being in the middle.

Of course, you can't do anything about where your tendons attach to the bones; however, this helps you understand why you and your training partners don't always progress at the same rate. Because many people get discouraged when their partners progress faster, it's good to know why not all arms were created equal. Other than the fact that everyone is different, here's the good news: lift diligently and intelligently, and you'll get stronger. In short, you'll be building the body you've always dreamed about.

Fiber Types

If you went to the lab to construct the perfect weightlifter, you'd use lots of fast-twitch muscle fibers (they're the kind capable of the greatest gains in size and strength), short arms and legs, and long tendons. When 6-footer Jonathan accompanied Deidre and her teammates to her powerlifting meets, he felt like Kareem Abdul-Jabbar at a jockey convention. At a bicycle race, he looks like one of the herd. (This may explain why he went into bicycle racing instead of competitive lifting.) Nevertheless, he lifts diligently to improve his cycling performance. On the other hand, Deidre, who carries 122 pounds of sculpted muscle on her 5-foot, 3-inch frame, has the ideal muscle type and body for hoisting prodigious amounts of weight. Did she have to train like a Trojan to become a world champion? Definitively yes. Could she have been a comparatively good cyclist or basketball player? Smart money says no.

FLEX FACTS

Some Eastern Bloc countries have been known to perform muscle biopsies on young children to determine whether they have predominantly fast-twitch or slow-twitch muscle fibers. This information allows them to direct the kids to sports that favor their particular physiological makeup.

Your next question might be: If you can't change these things, why even bother discussing them? For the simple fact that knowing about these variables can help prevent unnecessary frustration in the weight room. As we mentioned earlier, everyone can get stronger from weightlifting, but each person responds differently, even if the stimulus is the same.

Now that you know about some of the things you can't alter, let's talk about some of those you can. Luckily, regardless of your genetics, height, or body type, the body is an amazing machine that adapts beautifully when called upon. If you run a lot, your legs will respond; if you swim or kayak a lot, the upper body snaps to attention. The same is true of lifting weights: lift right and lift often, and the gains are there to be had.

Get with the Program

Although there are unyielding universal truths when it comes to developing a strength-training program, it's just common sense to tailor your routine to you—not some prototypical lifter who may have different goals, time constraints, and so forth.

Starting in Chapter 7, we give you a variety of exercises to work all your major muscle groups. Don't know how to awaken your dormant latissimus dorsi? No problem—we offer step-by-step instructions. And in Chapter 13, we give you suggestions about which exercises are most appropriate for you, given your specific goals. After all, if you want to improve your 10K running time, buffing up your biceps isn't time well spent. Strong hamstrings—well, that's a muscle of a different color.

For now, let's go over some of the fundamental aspects of a sound training routine.

What to Do?

For virtually every body part we discuss, we show you a few exercises. For every exercise we show you, there are usually at least two or three more—some good, some not so good—you could do instead. In most cases, these exercises are interchangeable. They're not really all that different. The most important point is to be sure you train all your major muscle groups, and train them in a logical order. Logical order? Yes. As we mentioned earlier, if, for example, you train your biceps first, your arms are likely to be too tired to offer proper assistance when you work your back or shoulders. As a rule, it's best to work the larger muscles first and work in descending size order. If you were going to hit all your major muscle groups on a particular day, you'd start with, say, your hips and legs and move down the list:

1. Hips and legs
2. Back
3. Chest
4. Shoulders
5. Biceps
6. Triceps
7. Abdominals

No, that's not written in stone—for instance, there's no real problem with switching the chest and the back or the biceps and the triceps—but it's a good guideline.

Schedule

When it comes to weightlifting, more is not always better. For instance, your initial temptation may be to take your ambitious mind and eager muscles to the gym as often as possible, but that strategy can actually work against you. Again, one essential key is to know when to work out and when to rest. Too much of one or the other, and you've upset the apple cart.

Keep in mind that, as you lift, you're actually fatiguing and wearing down the muscle tissue. It's during the recovery process that your muscles actually grow bigger and stronger. So never train the same muscles on consecutive days; it's actually counterproductive.

That's where a *split routine* comes in. In this program, you train different muscles on different days. So although you might lift on consecutive days—chest, shoulders, and triceps on Monday; legs, back, and biceps on Tuesday—you use different muscles each day. This gives you ample time for your muscles to recover and also means you'll be doing fewer exercises on any given day. This prevents burnout, allows you to spend less time lifting on each visit, and means you'll be able to work more intensely on the exercises you do. Don't sweat the particulars right now; we talk lots more about split routines in Chapter 13

DEFINITION

A **split routine** is a strength-training program in which you divide your body's muscles into two or more groups. On the first day of a split routine, you train muscle groups A and B; the following day, it's on to groups C and D.

At the other end of the "too many" spectrum, if you train too infrequently, you'll lose the strength gains you made in one session by the next. Even if you do the best routine in the world on January 1 and little or no training until February 1, the result will be minimal (at best) in the strength gains department. That should come as no surprise, but we hear people who lift twice a month lament the fact that they're not making much progress.

So what is the ideal frequency? That varies from individual to individual and has a lot to do with how hard each training session is. Here's another immutable rule to note: a hard workout requires more recovery time than an easy one.

Individual strengths and weaknesses aside, two workouts per week is good; three may be better. Whenever possible, we advise beginners to aim for three workouts. If you manage to do two, fine; however, if you're shooting for two, the tendency is that you'll miss one and compromise your gains. There's another reason three sessions may be better than two. Early in your workout life, one of our primary goals is to get your brain and body used to the exercises. At this stage, we're less concerned with intensity than frequency. So don't worry about your body's ability to tolerate three workouts a week. Once you make going to the gym a regular part of your life—when your weightlifting workout becomes part of your regular routine—you'll up the intensity and really start to see significant gains.

Reps

The repetition, or *rep*, is the basic unit of any weightlifting program. Think of each rep as a nail a carpenter uses to hammer the studs of a house. Although you need to know the big picture, the walls will fall down if you don't pay proper attention to which nail goes where. Unless you first focus on each and every rep, other variables, such as how many reps per set, how many sets per exercise, and the choice of exercise, don't really matter.

How Fast?

Because it's quite important to perform every rep with proper technique, let's do a quick rep check review.

A good guideline to follow while you're performing that perfect rep for most exercises is to count to 3 during the positive (or concentric) phase, hold for a count of 1, and count to 3 for the negative (or eccentric) phase. By controlling the speed, you accomplish a couple productive things:

- First and foremost, you maximize your safety and minimize the stress on your joints.

- You ensure that momentum is a nonfactor, which means you stress the muscles as much as possible and get the best bang for your buck.

- By keeping constant form for every rep of every workout, you're able to measure your progress.

For those of us who are goal oriented (which tends to be just about everyone who works out regularly) or those who just like to know that something is working, doing each rep as we just described is vital.

SPOT ME

A good way to gauge whether you're doing an exercise too fast is to try to stop at various points along the range of motion. If you're doing the exercise correctly, you should be able to stop on a dime without momentum carrying you farther than you want.

Consider the following scenario. On January 1, you do a biceps curl with 15-pound dumbbells and are able to do 11 repetitions in a 3-1-3 cadence with textbook-perfect form. If by March 1 you're up to 13 reps, with the same weight and form, clearly you have made progress. On the other hand, if you never pay any attention to anything other than how much weight you hoist and how many reps you've done, an increase in how many reps you do could be the result of changes in form rather than strength gains. This type of approach highlights our "lift to gain strength, not demonstrate strength" philosophy. It's not the best way to impress your musclehead friends in the gym, but it's a great way to get strong and healthy while staying injury free.

WEIGHT A MINUTE

It's important to perform each repetition in a slow, controlled fashion. This not only ensures that the exercise is effective, but it also minimizes the chance of orthopedic injury.

How Many Reps?

Now that we've established how you should perform each rep, let's examine how many reps you should do in each set. Walking around your local gym, you're likely to hear all sorts of different theories. Odds are that few, if any, are based on fact. Many will be based on refined analytical thinking that goes something like this: *Big Bob does sets of 25 for each exercise, and he's bigger than anybody else in the joint. That must be the way to go.* Or, *I read in a bodybuilding magazine that Ms. Olympia never does more than five reps per set, so that's what I'll do.* Again, how big and strong you get is largely a factor of genetics. Just because Bob the Bruiser is as broad as a barn door doesn't mean you will be, too. Some guys out there seemingly get big just by looking at a dumbbell rack.

Wander around the gym a little longer, and you're also likely to hear another bit of misinformation that goes something like this: using high weight with low reps builds bulk, but low weight and high reps helps build definition. Sometimes people will even tell you that lifting like that will actually elongate the muscle. Not so!

Here's the scoop. First of all, despite what you may hear from misguided trainers or in Pilates class, your muscle isn't going to get any longer by lifting weights—it attaches to a tendon, which attaches to a bone, and that's that. As for the notion that high reps define or tone your muscles more than low reps, wrong again. No medical facts substantiate such a statement. Too many other factors, such as genetics and nutrition, come into play—and besides, intensity, not the number of reps, makes most of the difference.

Where this supposedly correct fact came from, we don't know. Perhaps it derives from the fact that a long set often produces a burning sensation in your muscles—flash back to Jane Fonda in a leotard encouraging you to "feel the burn"—but that burn doesn't indicate that fat is being burned. Muscles look defined when there's a minimal layer of fat covering them. It's as simple as that. So the question remains: How many reps should you do? For most exercises, a range of 10 to 12 repetitions at a 3-second, pause, 3-second cadence is appropriate. When you can perform more than 12 well-executed reps at a given weight, it's time to up the weight by about 5 percent. The last rep of the set should always be a challenge—a noble effort we refer to as elegant failure.

FLEX FACTS

Muscular fatigue and a burning sensation during strenuous exercise are often due to a high concentration of lactic acid, which accumulates in the blood when the energy demands of an exercise exceed the supply or utilization rate of oxygen.

How Many Sets?

Once again, ask five so-called experts about the optimal number of reps to do, and you're likely to get five different answers. In fact, this question produces quite a bit of controversy—controversy, we must add, that's based on fiction rather than on fact.

Traditionally, lifters have performed two or three sets per exercise, although often you hear about people doing as many as five or six. However, if you read the many studies on the subject, most of them seem to indicate that one set (yes, one set!) can be just as effective as and far more efficient than doing multiple sets. By "effective," we mean that you can get every bit as strong. By "efficient," we mean that you can gain strength in a fraction of the time. If you use that extra time to do your cardiovascular training, to stretch, or to practice your sport, you're upping your fitness quotient twofold.

When Jonathan warmed the bench for his junior varsity basketball team at Hunter College, he observed many of the varsity players spending several hours a day in the weight room. Although they got plenty strong, they also shot a measly 65 percent from the foul line. Those players probably would have been much better served by cutting their lifting time in half and practicing their shooting.

Now, we're not saying that you can't or won't get strong from two, three, or more sets per exercise—of course, you will. We're just saying that you can get nearly as strong (if not every bit as strong) from one set, too. At the very least, doing one set is far more efficient than doing multiple sets. Again, whether you do 1 set or 10, the most important point to keep in mind is that the last repetition of any set should be difficult. That's why it's important to avoid what we call the magic number syndrome. This occurs when people stop at a given number of reps (usually 10, 12, or 15) even though they've got a lot of gas left in the tank. If you reach your tenth rep and you can do another rep or two without sacrificing form or safety, do it. Remember that you're not a Swiss watch, but an evolving work in progress.

How Much Weight?

How much weight should you lift? This question is probably asked more than any other question in weightlifting.

Now that we've established that a range of 10 to 12 reps is ideal for most exercises, we need to find the weight that will allow you to do that many without compromising your form. As we said before, early on, your goal is to learn to do the exercises with the proper technique. In this initial phase of your lifting life, you should err on the side of caution when picking a weight to start with. Generally, the larger the muscle, the more weight you can handle. And as you'll quickly learn, you can move more weight with your legs than with your arms.

In Chapter 7, we begin to give you step-by-step instructions on how to actually perform these exercises. When you get started with each of them, begin with the lightest weight possible. If it's a machine, set it to one plate, to get the feel for it, and then add a little more. Right now, we want you to focus on technique without worrying about completing the lift. For exercises that require dumb-bells, use relatively light ones to accomplish the same aim. And for exercises with a barbell, try using the Olympic bar without weight—or even a lighter one, if necessary.

In any event, be sure not to strain or push too hard during your first few workouts. When you get the feel of things, you can gradually start to increase the weight during the next few workouts. Be patient. Increase the weight a little each time until you find a weight that will be challenging by the 10th or 11th rep. When you've found that weight, stay with it until you can do 12 good reps. When you can do 12 solid reps without straining a vital organ, it's time to increase the weight. When you bump up the weight, try for about a 5 percent increase. Adding that extra weight should make reaching 10 a challenge again.

Here's another issue to keep in mind: if you've been lifting for six months and find that you're unable to perform 12 reps even though you did so last week, don't worry. The key is form, concentration, and intensity. As long as you reach elegant failure on your 9th, 10th, or 11th rep, you're making progress. Lack of sleep, stress, and myriad other factors impact how you feel on any given day, so cut yourself some slack as long as you're working hard.

How Much Rest?

The amount of rest to take between exercises is as fundamental a concern as any other, but for some reason, it is the one issue often overlooked. For example, most gym veterans can tell you how much weight they use and how many reps they do for any exercise, but few pay much attention to how much rest they take between sets.

From a physiological point of view, there's no real reason to take more than 3 minutes between sets. By that time, your ATP (remember, ATP is your body's source of immediate energy) is about 99 percent replenished and your body is as ready as it's going to be. From a practical point of view, there's no reason for a beginning lifter to wait that long between sets. Two minutes gives your muscles ample time to recover and gives a workout partner time to change the weight and do a set without wasting undue time.

We don't want to make working out a stressful bit of time management, but be aware that when you're not thinking about time, 2 minutes flies by. In fact, very often people have brief chats between sets that last anywhere from 4 to 15 minutes. Ask them how long they take between sets, and they assume that it's only a few minutes. Before you know it, the workout that should take you 45 minutes to an hour has stretched to 1½ hours. Early on, at least, it's good to time yourself between sets. After you find a rhythm, your body will know the appropriate amount of rest to take.

Spotter, Please

Remember, a spotter is someone who is ready to help the lifter in case he or she can't complete a lift. As someone who has chosen to lift a heavy object—often over your precious head or neck—it's your responsibility to be sure you have a spotter whenever you're doing an exercise that may jeopardize your health and welfare. Probably the two most important exercises to have a spotter for when you're using free weights are the squat (see Chapter 7) and the bench press (see Chapter 9), but they're not the only ones. Again, if you can't lift the weight, you're in serious trouble.

Even when you're using a machine or doing free weight exercises and your safety isn't jeopardized by the absence of a spotter, a helping hand can help you get more out of an exercise.

How? We all have exercises we find particularly difficult. Let's say that, for you, it's shoulder presses. (For an illustration, see Chapter 10.) Often just having someone stand next to you provides the extra motivation to focus and finish the set with good form and maximum effort. Also, a spotter can help you get a few extra reps out of any exercise by offering the barest assistance. We've had spotters provide invaluable help simply by nudging the weight with two fingers.

As the lifter, it's your responsibility to tell the spotter what you're going to do. Let him or her know how many reps you're hoping to do, whether you want a spot on the lift-off (when you first pick the weight off the stand), and so on. It's also your job to never give up on a lift. Jonathan has helped spot powerlifters bench pressing more than 400 pounds. He couldn't lift close to that much by himself, but as long as the lifter doesn't bail out on the lift, he'll never have to. In fact, even if the bruising powerlifter can't moose out that last rep, as long as he gives it his best effort, Jonathan has to help with only the last few pounds.

Sooner or later, you'll be asked to switch places and act as a spotter. In that case, it's your job to ensure the lifter's safety. Here's the key: never agree to do something you can't. And if you're not sure what's expected of you, ask. A good spotter is like a good baseball umpire—as unobtrusive as possible. Aside from an inattentive one, an overanxious spotter is the next biggest sinner. After you've ensured that the lifter doesn't drop 200 pounds on his esophagus, the spotter's job is to be sure the weight keeps moving with as little assistance as possible. Remember, you're doing the lifter a disservice if you provide too much assistance.

If you see the weight stop moving, give it a little nudge. (On most exercises that use a barbell, you're usually best off lifting the bar itself. In the case of exercises that use dumbbells, it's usually preferable to nudge the lifter's elbows.) After you've done it a few times, you'll get the hang of it. The most important points to keep in mind are to always pay attention, avoid jumping in too soon, and stay close enough to the lifter to help when needed.

Now that you understand the various x-factors of weight training, let's move on and learn some specific exercises.

The Least You Need to Know

- Understanding why no two lifters are alike should clear up a lot of questions and alleviate any frustration you may feel.
- The anatomy of a repetition is of the utmost importance.
- The nitty-gritty of a strength-training program includes how many reps, how many sets, and how much weight.
- Offering assistance to your fellow lifters is a standard part of gym etiquette.

The Legs

In This Chapter

- Understanding what's what
- Building your legs with two great free weight exercises
- Getting buffer gams with seven leg-machine exercises

Okay, anatomy fans. What's the largest group of muscles in your body? Lats? Wrong. Pecs? Nope. Abdominals? Sorry. In fact, the largest muscles you have are located below your waist. When most people think of their legs, they think of the muscles in two major groups: upper and lower, or thighs and calves. Of course, there's a lot more going on in those sturdy legs of yours. So that you know what we're talking about when we recommend the exercises that follow, here's a quick tour of Leg World.

One of these muscle groups is the *gluteus maximus*, or glutes, a wide band of muscle that covers your entire butt area. If you've ridden a horse too long or cycled for hours at a time, these are the muscles that doth protest too much. They are also the muscles that are featured in all those salacious jeans ads. The glutes, of course, can do more than sell pants. Their primary function is to extend your legs from your hips when your leg is bent—in other words, when you're running for the bus.

Located opposite your glutes are your *hip flexors*. Although several muscles contribute to the act of hip flexion, the largest is called the *iliopsoas*. These muscles don't receive much attention. In fact, in all our years of going to the gym, we've never heard someone say, "Hey, nice iliopsoas." (We think this is a shame, but there's not much we can do about it.)

The iliopsoas is a strong muscle that doesn't usually need much concentrated work because it receives quite a bit of work on a daily basis from walking, running, and climbing stairs. In fact, because we tend to sit so much, it is the muscle that is often too tight. As a result, this muscle is usually better served by being stretched than by being strengthened. If it becomes too tight, this tricky muscle that runs from the lumbar spine to the inside of the uppermost part of the long bone in the thigh (femur) can pull your pelvis forward and put stress on your lumbar spine. The result? Serious lower-back pain.

On the sides of your hips are the hip abductors, the main one being the *gluteus medius*. This muscle works to move your leg away from your body—while pushing off during inline skating, for example. Their companions, located on the inner part of the thigh, are the adductors, which draw your leg toward your body.

The big boys in the band are the *quadriceps*, or quads. These muscles span the entire front part of your leg. If you're an NFL running back or a professional cyclist, odds are, your quads are like large loaves of bread. The quads are comprised of four muscles (hence the name *quad*riceps) that work to straighten your lower leg from a bent position. One of them, the *rectus femoris*, crosses the hip joint and works to bend as well as flex the hip.

Opposite the quadriceps are your *hamstrings*, which cover the entire posterior aspect of your upper leg. The hamstrings are actually three muscles that work in concert to perform two actions: to extend your leg from your hip when your leg is straight and to bend your lower leg from the straight position.

Finally, your calves are the muscles located near the bottom of your legs. One of them is the gastrocnemius (or gastroc). This diamond-shaped muscle works to push you up on your toes. The other muscle, the soleus, is deeper and comes into play when your knees are bent and you need to lift your heel. The third muscle, located on your shin in the front of your leg, is called the tibialis anterior. This is the muscle that rears its ugly head when you come down with a case of shin splints. It functions to lift your toes from the floor. Think back to when you were speeding down the highway and saw flashing lights in your rearview mirror. The muscle that pulls your lead foot off the gas pedal is the tibialis anterior. In fact, the next time you're stopped by a cop for speeding, tell the officer you have chronically tight tibialis anteriors. If that doesn't work, hope you have a pregnant woman in the car.

What's the Point?

We hear comments like these all the time: "I'm a swimmer—why do I need strong leg muscles?" Or "I cycle a lot, so I don't need to work my legs." Or "I'm a runner and don't want to do leg exercises because my legs will get too big"—or any number of other faulty lines of reasoning.

Here are good reasons lifting weights with your legs will serve you well:

- Strong leg muscles are the key to injury prevention in sports from cycling to running. In fact, weak leg muscles and muscle imbalances are the primary reasons runners are unable to complete proper training for a marathon.

- Strong legs help your performance on the field. For example, some people think a baseball pitcher can throw a baseball nearly 100 miles per hour because he has an exceptional arm. Of course he does, but much of his power is generated by his powerful hips and thighs.

- Strong muscles protect your hip, knee, and ankle joints from a lifetime of stress—from running, jumping, and going up and down stairs.

- Your legs will look good when you wear shorts. Similarly, just think about how weird it looks to have a great upper body and itty-bitty legs.

- For the elderly, keeping the legs strong is important for balance, walking moderate to long distances, and moving from a sitting to a standing position.

Now that we've convinced you that you need strong legs, let's show you how to get them.

Many of the lower-body exercises we recommend for you to get started with use machines; however, two free weight exercises can contribute to an extremely effective lower-body routine. These exercises—the squat and the lunge—involve not only your legs, but your entire body, to stabilize you during the performance of the lift. Oh yeah, one sobering note: both are difficult.

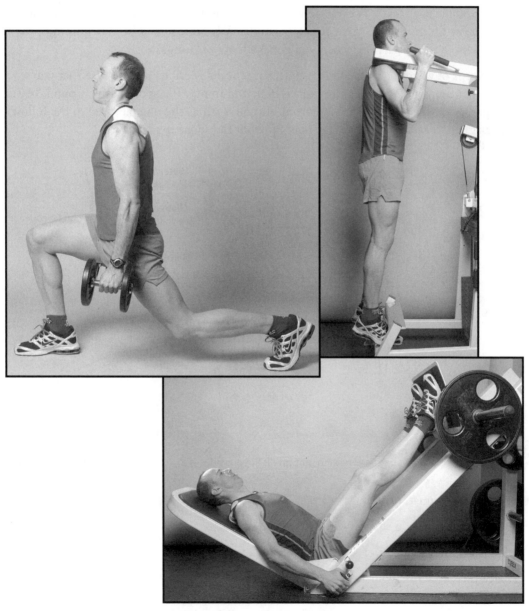

Some of the exercises in this chapter.

Squat

Ah, the beloved and dreaded squat. The squat, a lower-body exercise that requires you to shoulder a barbell and literally squat, is a great way to strengthen your legs. When the 122-pound Deidre was powerlifting at the world class level, she was able to do eight repetitions with 185 pounds. In competition, her personal record was 330 pounds. Although no sane person (at least, no sane 122-pound person) will attempt to do that much weight, the point is that squatting is a demanding exercise. Despite its incredible payback, it is extremely important that you pay strict attention to your form—and that you never lift more than you can safely handle. We omit squats from beginning programs, but we keep them in the arsenal for when you get the hang of things.

A few other words of warning: work with a spotter whenever possible, and be sure that you're warmed up. Squatting when your legs are stiff is courting injury. If a spotter isn't around, be sure to use an apparatus that's designed for squatting. A cage, such as the one pictured in the following figures, is designed to catch you if you can't get up from the squatting position.

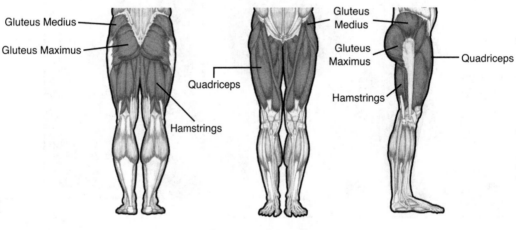

Squat: muscles used.

FLEX FACTS

Squats have many variations. Holding dumbbells at your sides is a great one and doesn't require a spotter.

When performing a squat, **don't:**

- Lean forward as you squat.
- Squat without a spotter or safety rack.
- Place the bar across your neck.

SPOT ME

Although some trainers consider it safer to do a *quarter-squat,* where you bend to only about 45°, we question whether that's the case. When you cut the range of motion that far, there's a tendency to greatly increase the weight used, which puts much more stress on your back.

Do:

- Keep your abdominals tight.
- Keep your weight on your heels, not on your toes.
- Maintain an upright posture.
- Place the bar across your upper back.

Here's how you properly perform a squat:

1. Stand underneath the barbell with your feet slightly wider than shoulder width apart.

2. With your arms holding the barbell with a grip about 6 to 8 inches from your shoulders, lift the barbell off the rack.

3. Take one step backward so you don't hit the racks as you squat, and keep your toes pointed slightly outward.

4. Keeping your back straight, begin to bend your knees until your thighs are parallel to the floor. Don't squat deeper. However, if you squat too little, you're not maximizing the benefits of the exercise—remember that a greater range of motion ensures full strength gains.

5. Return to your starting position.

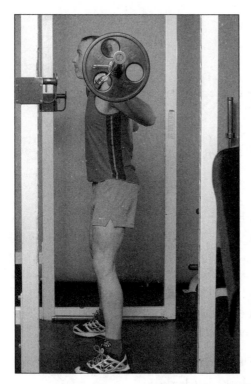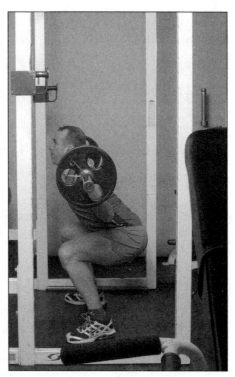

Squat start/finish position (left). Squat middle position (right).

Lunge

Lunges use the same muscles squats do. However, you don't need nearly as much weight because you're exercising one leg at a time. Lunges also require more concentration. Space out, and you're likely to lose your balance. Whether you do lunges or squats is a personal preference; you don't need to do both. Deidre eschews lunges because she'd rather get both legs done at the same time. Because Jonathan has a strength deficit between his right and left legs, he does them a lot more for the left leg.

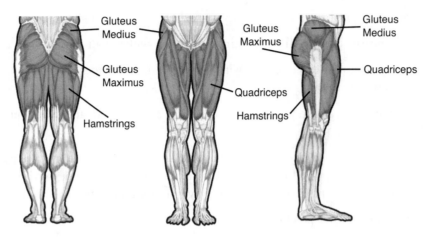

Lunge: muscles used.

When performing a lunge, **don't**:

- Lean forward.
- Let your knee pass forward of your big toe in the middle position.

Do:

- Keep your abdominals tight and your back straight.
- Keep your torso upright.

Keep in mind that you can also do this exercise with a barbell.

Here's how you properly perform a lunge:

1. While holding a dumbbell in each hand (with your palms facing your outer thighs), stand with your feet slightly less than shoulder width apart.

2. Now move your right leg approximately one stride length in front of your left. The exercise is called a *lunge* but is more aptly named a *controlled lunge*.

3. Bend your right and left knees until your right thigh is parallel to the ground.

4. Return to the starting position. Repeat with the left leg.

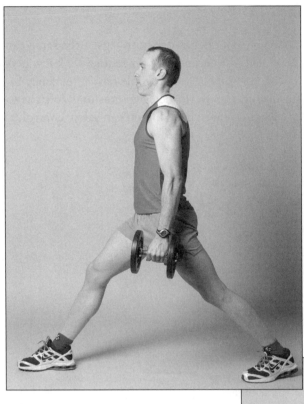

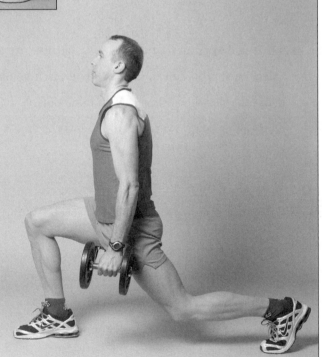

Lunge start/finish position (top). Lunge middle position (bottom).

Leg Press

The leg press machine is one of our favorites because you can safely work both legs at the same time even while using a lot of weight. However, don't be fooled just because it's a machine; we know people who have injured both their back and their ribs. How? For some reason, people have a tendency to load on the weight. Stacking on too many big plates brings the overloaded sled crashing down as soon as they release the brake. The obvious point? Don't add more weight than you can safely control for 10 to 12 repetitions.

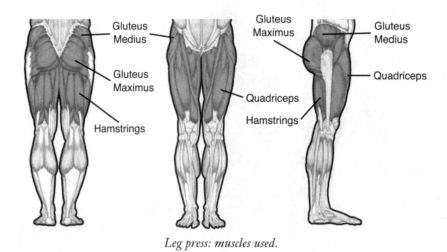

Leg press: muscles used.

The keys to a safe workout on the leg-press machine are as follows:

- Select an appropriate amount of weight that you can safely do on your own.
- Bring the sled down slowly. Maintain control.
- Don't allow your lower back to rise off the seat pad. If this happens, you are bringing your knees too close to your chest.

WEIGHT A MINUTE

This exercise may be contraindicated for people with hyperextended (excessive backward bend) knees.

When performing a leg press, **don't:**

- Lock or snap your knees at the top of the movement.
- Arch your back.
- Allow your buttocks to lift off the seat.

Do:

- Keep your abdominals tight.
- Bear weight on the midfoot to heel portion of your feet, not your toes.

Here's how you properly perform a leg press:

1. Position yourself on the machine and place your feet on the sled at approximately shoulder width apart.

2. Point your toes outward slightly.

3. Grasp the handles on either side of the seat.

4. Disengage the brake, and slowly lower the sled until your knees are bent to 90° or until your lower back comes off the sled.

5. Pause and slowly return to the starting position.

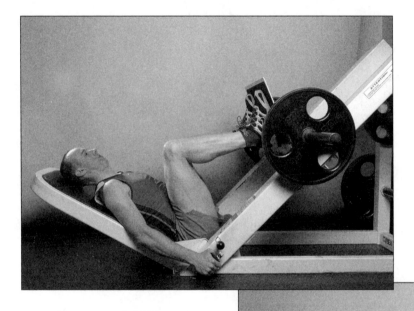

Leg press start/finish position (top). Leg press middle position (bottom).

Leg Extensions

Want quads like Lance Armstrong's? Do leg extensions. (Of course, it would help if you rode a bicycle 500 miles a week.) Okay, perhaps you won't build the legs of a Tour de France champion, but done diligently, leg extensions are among the best ways to build powerful upper thighs. Be very careful not to do more weight than you can handle for 10 solid repetitions. If you overdo it on this machine, you could end up with patellar tendinitis (an inflammation of the tendon just below the knee, caused by overuse). And if you've had anterior cruciate ligament (ACL) reconstruction or other knee surgery, you probably want to avoid leg extensions.

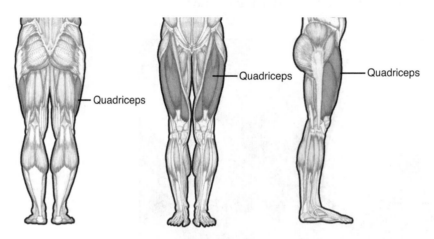

Leg extension: muscles used.

When performing a leg extension, **don't:**

- Jerk your legs up rapidly.
- Allow the weights being lifted to slam down against the weight stack between repetitions.
- Lock or snap your legs straight.
- Swing your trunk back and forth.

Do:

- Keep your back against the back pad.
- Focus on your quads.

Here's how you properly perform a leg extension:

1. Sit with your back against the back pad, and position your shins behind the lower leg pad.

2. Grasp the handles on either side of the seat.

3. Straighten your lower legs as high as possible.

4. Return under control to the initial starting position.

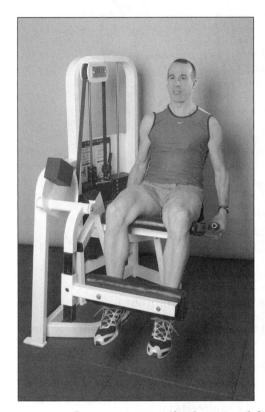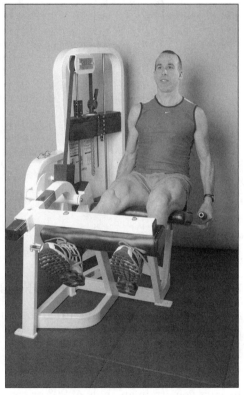

Leg extension start/finish position (left). Leg extension middle position (right).

Leg Curls

Leg curls are to your hamstrings what leg extensions are to your quads. Because muscular balance is so essential, it's important to build both your quads and your hams so that one doesn't overwhelm the other. Again, remember to stretch your hamstrings before doing this exercise.

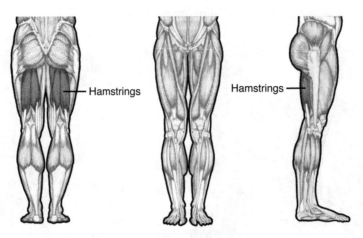

Leg curls: muscles used.

When performing a leg curl, **don't:**

- Arch your back or lift your pelvis.
- Lie with your head in the left- or right-side position. Rest on your forehead.
- Allow the weight stack being lifted to slam down on the remaining weight stack between repetitions.

Do:

- Be sure you attain an angle of 90° or less at the midposition.
- Keep your hips on the bench.

WEIGHT A MINUTE

Leg curls are not recommended for people with low-back pain or hyperextended knees. Some gyms have a leg curl machine on which you sit rather than lie down, and it's more appropriate for people suffering from back pain. If you have hyperextended knees, a standing leg curl machine is better for you. If you don't have these options, do the following: for lower-back pain, place towels beneath your abdomen to support your back. For hyperextended knees, adjust the rotary arm so that your knees are slightly bent.

Here's how you properly perform a leg curl:

1. Lie face down on the bench and place your lower legs underneath the roller pads.

2. Keep the tops of your kneecaps positioned just over the edge of the bench pad, not on the pad itself.

3. Grasp the handles on either side of the bench.

4. Pull up your heels as close to your buttocks as possible.

5. Slowly return to the initial starting position.

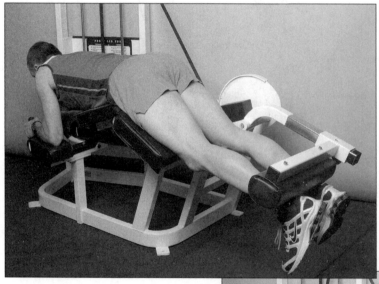

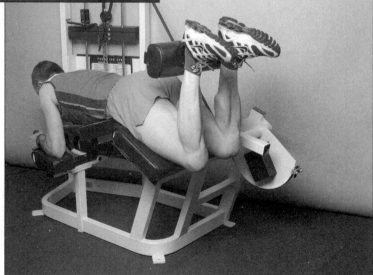

Leg curl start/finish position (top). Leg curl middle position (bottom).

Calf Raises (Standing)

Much of your ability to continue to do even the most basic activities is due to muscular endurance. Muscular endurance is related to muscular strength. If you want to continue to walk up stairs with a spring in your step, you'd better begin to strengthen those gastroc muscles.

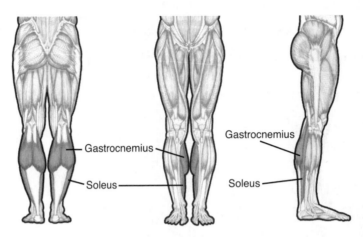

Standing calf raise: muscles used.

When performing a standing calf raise, **don't:**

- Arch your back.
- Rock back and forth.
- Perform the exercise rapidly.

Do:

- Keep your abdominals tight and your back erect.
- Keep your legs straight.
- If it burns, you're doing it right.

Here's how you properly perform a standing calf raise:

1. Stand on the bottom step so that the balls of your feet are on the edge of the step and your heels extend over the edge.

2. Position your shoulders beneath the pads, and place your hands on either side of the pads.

3. Keeping your legs straight, rise onto your toes as high as possible.

4. Return slowly to a position where your heels are hanging down as far as possible. This ensures a good stretch.

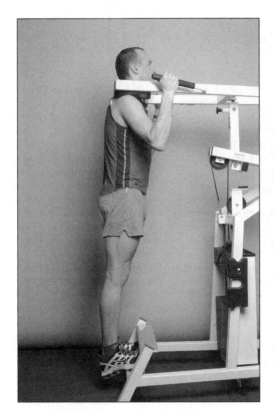 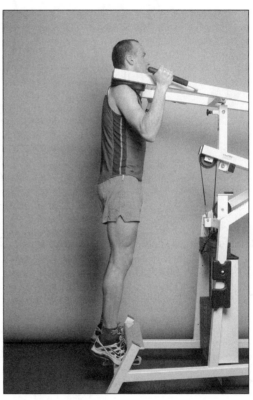

Standing calf raise start/finish position (left). Standing calf raise middle position (right).

Calf Raises (Seated)

As we explained earlier, the soleus muscle is engaged while the knee is bent. It follows that the way to strengthen this muscle is to do so while the knees are bent. This muscle is extremely important, especially if you're a runner. It is a deep muscle (located close to your lower leg bone) that's called into play with endurance activities. If these muscles are weak, they fatigue and can become extremely painful.

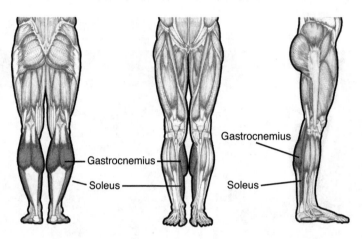

Seated calf raise: muscles used.

When performing a seated calf raise, **don't:**

- Rock back and forth.
- Perform the exercise rapidly.

Do:

- Keep your abdominals tight and your back erect.
- Remember, burn, baby, burn.

Here's how you properly perform a seated calf raise:

1. Sit on the seat with your knees under the pads.

2. Position the balls of your feet on the edge of the foot plate.

3. Disengage the brake, allowing your heels to hang over the edge.

4. Rise up on your toes as high as possible.

5. Return slowly to a position where your heels are hanging down as far as possible, to ensure a good stretch.

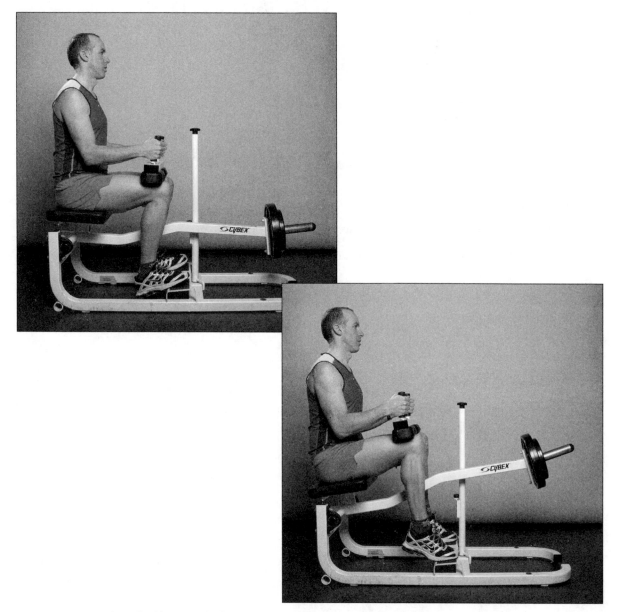

Seated calf raise start/finish position (top). Seated calf raise middle position (bottom).

Hip Abduction

Because our muscles don't work in a vacuum, you don't really need to isolate your hip abductor muscles. They're already busy stabilizing and working while you're performing exercises such as squats and lunges. However, there's no harm done if you choose to isolate these muscles.

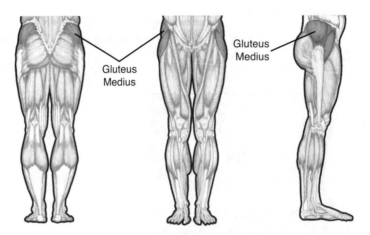

Gluteus Medius

Gluteus Medius

Hip abduction: muscles used.

When performing a hip abduction, **don't**:

- Bend forward as you perform the exercise.

- Allow the weight stack to slam down on the remaining weight stack between repetitions.

Do:

- Keep your abdominals tight and your back erect.

- Keep your head and trunk against the back pad.

SPOT ME

People with relatively short legs may require an additional back pad for this exercise.

Here's how you properly perform a hip abduction:

1. Sit on the machine with your back against the back pad and your outer legs against the thigh pads.

2. Secure the belt, if there is one.

3. Push your legs apart as far as possible by pushing against the thigh pads.

4. Return slowly to the initial starting position.

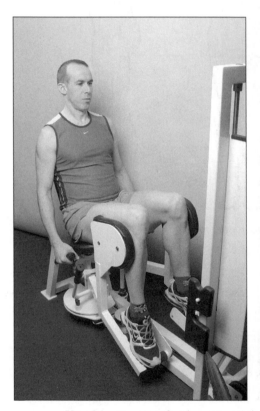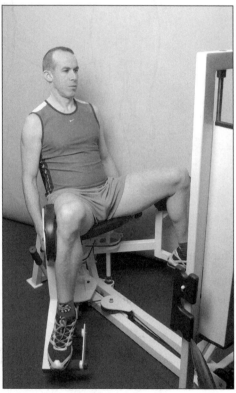

Hip abduction start/finish position (left). Hip abduction middle position (right).

Hip Adduction

Our muscles are not islands unto themselves; your adductors are working in conjunction with other muscles while doing squats, leg presses, or lunges. However, if you are involved in a sport that over-stretches and/or overuses the adductors, you will definitely need to isolate them with these exercises. When Deidre powerlifted, she developed adductor tendonitis in both legs because she constantly overstretched her adductors with her wide-stance deadlifts.

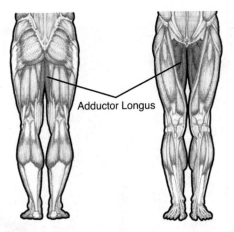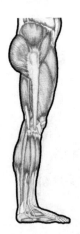

Adductor Longus

Hip adduction: muscles used.

When performing a hip adduction, **don't:**

- Allow the weight stack being lifted to slam down on the remaining weight stack between repetitions.

Do:

- Keep your abdominals tight and your back erect.
- Keep your head and trunk against the back pad.

Don't be surprised to see people (usually women) doing hundreds of reps of abduction and adduction exercises, in the hope of burning fat and slimming their thighs. The problem is that when a muscle works hard enough it gets bigger, not smaller. (Those guys doing biceps curls all day aren't trying to get their arms to shrink!) Furthermore, the muscle that's exercising has nothing to do with where fat is burned. So although there are reasons to work these muscles, shrinking your thighs isn't one of them.

Here's how you properly perform a hip adduction:

1. Sit on the machine with your back against the back pad and your inner legs against the thigh pads.

2. Secure the belt, if there is one.

3. Bring your legs together as close as possible by pushing against the thigh pads.

4. Return slowly to the initial starting position.

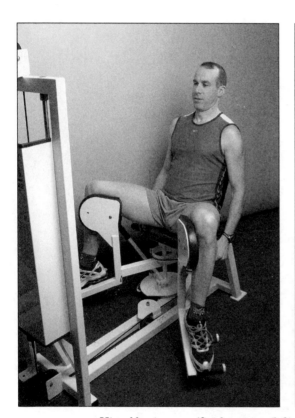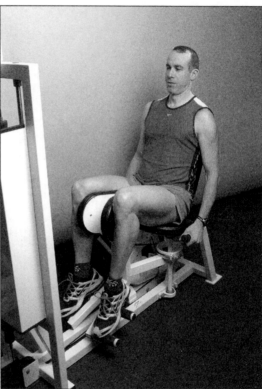

Hip adduction start/finish position (left). Hip adduction middle position (right).

The Back

In This Chapter

- Developing lats for that V shape
- Supporting your back to avoid injury
- Keeping your posture

Latissimus dorsi (or lats) are what gives us that V shape—that rear view bystanders get to admire while we stare straight ahead. The lats are broad muscles that span the area from just behind each armpit to the center of your lower back. These muscles are key for hoisting yourself up while rock climbing, rowing, and performing pull-ups—to name just a few.

For men, large lats provide that wide expanse of muscle that resembles the top of a manta ray. Many women who weight-train notice that well-developed lats offer the illusion that their waist is narrower. In fact, it's not; it only appears that way, but few women we know complain about this complimentary illusion.

Just above the lats are the *trapezius* muscles (or traps). These powerful muscles run from just below the back of your skull to the edge of your shoulders, and down through the center of your back. When you shrug your shoulders, you're using your traps.

What else is going on in that back of yours? The *rhomboids*—major and minor—span the area between your spine and your shoulder blades. Along with your traps, the rhomboids retract, or squeeze your shoulder blades together. The rhomboids are shaped like a Christmas tree and are attached to the innermost part of your shoulder blades (scapula). Any exercise that brings the shoulder blades together works these muscles.

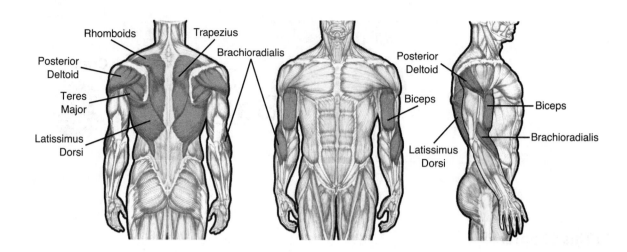

Why Bother?

Aside from looking good, strong back muscles are important for maintaining good posture, and vice versa. In other words, good posture equals a strong healthy back, and a strong back contributes to good posture. Slouching overstretches the muscles, making them work harder during the day. Because overworked muscles fatigue and often spasm, keeping your muscles at their proper working length and strength prevents this (again, assuming that you pay attention to your posture).

Here are three other reasons to train your back:

- Strong upper-back muscles enable you to maintain an erect sitting posture without fatigue. Slouching, a bad habit that accounts for untold amounts of chronic back pain, puts these muscles in an overstretched position. This weakens them and leads to muscle spasms, headaches, and backaches.

- Strong lats can help you scale that rock wall or give you more power while on the rowing machine, while in a swimming pool, or as you paddle a canoe or kayak.

- Strong upper-back muscles prevent muscle strength imbalances and protect the shoulders, especially in sports such as swimming, tennis, and pitching, which emphasize the anterior shoulders and pectoralis muscles.

The lats, being so large and expansive, respond well to both free weights and machines. As a matter of fact, you can probably work them much harder with machines than with free weights because you're able to use a little more weight and don't have to concentrate on form quite as much. However, using both is still important, especially when you concentrate on the smaller back muscles such as the rhomboids.

Following are a number of exercises that help develop both overall strength and specific back strength.

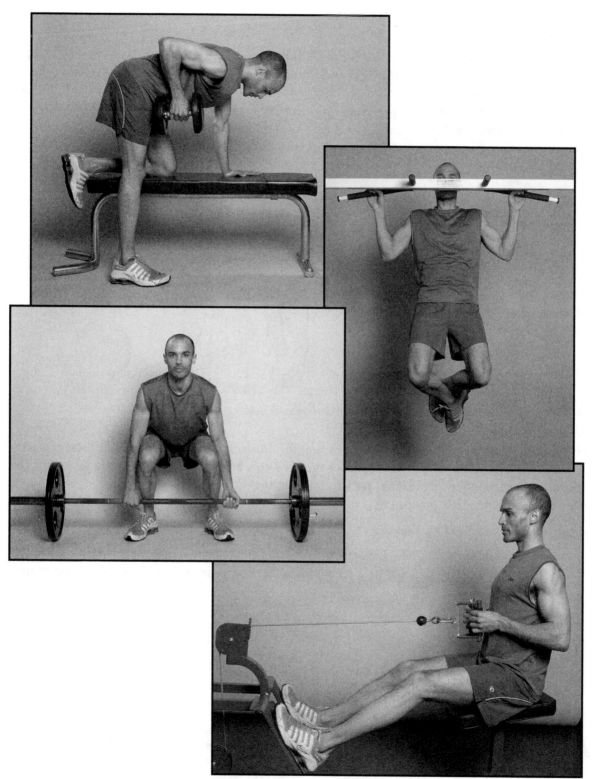

Some of the exercises in this chapter.

Deadlifts

One of the three powerlifting exercises, the deadlift is a good news/bad news deal. First the good news: the deadlift is one of the best overall body exercises you can do. Every muscle is involved during the deadlift: upper back, hips, quads, hamstrings, abdominals—you name it. Now the bad news: it's a challenging lift and must be performed with perfect form, or you'll risk injury. We omit it from beginning programs, but it can become a valuable weapon in your back-training arsenal as your strength training progresses.

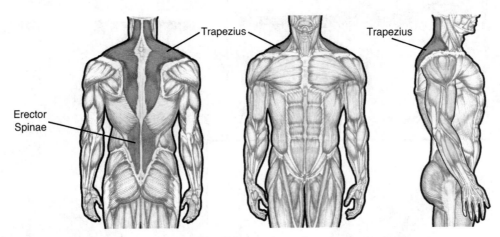

Deadlift: muscles used.

The most important point to keep in mind during this lift is that you must hold your back as erect as possible. Never allow your chest to go over the bar—this brings your body forward as you lift the weight, causing you to use your lower back for most of the lift instead of using your hips and legs. As you pull the weight, think of pushing your feet through the floor so you really get your legs into it.

When performing a deadlift, **don't:**

- Lift your hips too quickly. This transfers most of the effort to your lower back. Your legs, hips, and lower back should be working together, with your legs and hips doing most of the work.

- Snap or lock your knees as you straighten your legs.

- Lean back excessively.

- Bounce the weight off the floor between repetitions.

WEIGHT A MINUTE

Don't attempt this exercise if you have lower-back problems. People with long torsos often have difficulty performing this lift because the lower back becomes the pivot point.

Do:

- Keep your abdominals tight and your back as erect as possible.

- Keep your shoulder blades pulled together—this helps keep your back erect.

SPOT ME

When deadlifting with 45-pound plates, the bar begins just below your knees. The problem is that most people must learn the exercise with significantly less weight than that, which lowers the bar and increases how far you need to bend to get the bar. Start off using dumbbells instead of a barbell, to avoid back strain associated with bending too far.

Here's how you properly perform a deadlift:

1. Place your feet slightly wider apart than shoulder width.

2. Reach down and grasp the bar on the outside of the legs with a *reverse grip*.

DEFINITION

In the alternating grip or **reverse grip**, you hold the bar with the fingers of one hand facing your body and the fingers of your other hand facing away from your body. This improves your ability to hold the bar without it slipping out of your hands.

3. Lower your hips until your thighs are nearly parallel to the floor.

4. Flatten your lower back and look up slightly.

5. Be sure your weight is on your heels, not your toes. Form is of the utmost importance here, so be sure the first time you do this awesome lift that you do it with just the bar.

6. Stand upright by straightening your legs and upper body; pause and then slowly return to the initial starting position. Think of yourself as a piston or as an arrow being shot out of the bow.

7. Look up toward the ceiling, because that's where you want to go. (Typically, your body goes where your head and eyes go.) If you look straight ahead, you may come out of the lift going forward. Look up, and you'll usually come out going up.

8. As you lower the bar to the starting position, be sure to keep the bar close to your shins. In fact, the bar should actually graze your shins throughout the lift.

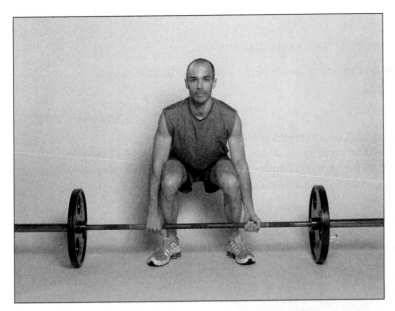

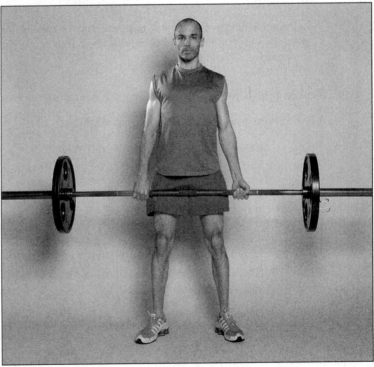

Deadlift start/finish position (top). Deadlift middle position (bottom).

Pull-ups and Chin-ups

If we were in jail and could have just one apparatus, we'd pine for a pull-up/chin-up bar. These simple exercises, which happen to be uncommonly difficult, are (along with the push-up and sit-up) very effective exercises when your access to equipment is limited. Here's the skinny on pull-ups: don't try once or twice and give up. Pull-ups and chin-ups are hard for nearly everyone, so don't get discouraged. If you stick with it, you'll improve rapidly because it's such a thorough strength-building exercise. The keys are effort and focus.

If weak arms and gravity have got you down, try doing an assisted chin-up or pull-up on a machine that allows you to lift only a percentage of your body weight. The *Gravitron* was the first of this type and is still the most popular, but gyms today have many others. To use these machines, you stand on a platform that pushes up to help you hoist your body weight. The directions are fairly simple, the rough equivalent of getting candy out of a vending machine—only much better for you.

FLEX FACTS

The Gravitron machine allows users to select either a percentage of their body weight or an amount of plated weight to assist them with the pull-up/chin-up. For example, if you weigh 150 pounds, you can set the machine to give you 50 percent assistance with the exercise, so you'd be pulling or chinning 75 pounds. Alternatively, you can select plated weights to give you 70 pounds of assistance.

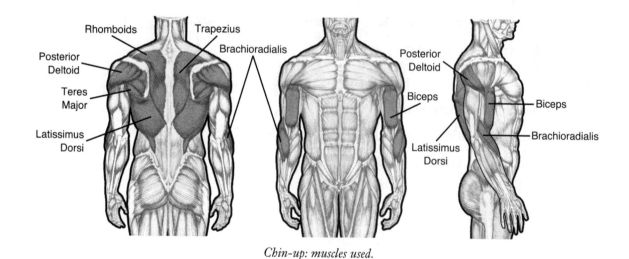

Chin-up: muscles used.

Here's how effective this exercise can be. Because a strong back is essential for a kayak paddler, Joe regularly does pull-ups as part of his strength-training regimen. (In fact, most paddlers do.) For years, he and a mate were running neck-and-neck in virtually every marathon race they did. However, one season Joe's paddling mate began whipping him regularly on the water. The difference? His friend had gone on a mad pull-up crusade, doing 20 sets of 10 repetitions regularly while Joe watched late-night TV.

Sound like a lot? It is. However, Joe has another friend who can do 100 consecutive pull-ups. This amazing specimen has a back as wide as a barn door and happens to be one of the best paddlers in Australia.

FLEX FACTS

At age 63, South Korea's Lee Chin-Yong holds the world record of 370 consecutive pull-ups. Not impressed? Robert Chisnail performed a record 22 consecutive one-armed pull-ups on a gymnastics ring!

Adhering to a regular pull-up regimen will have a major impact on your lats.

Concentrating on your breathing is extremely helpful. Remember on the positive or upward phase to exhale smoothly; reverse on the way down.

SPOT ME

The difference between the pull-up and the chin-up is the hand position. For pull-ups, palms face away from the body. For chin-ups, palms face toward the body. The underhand grip tends to stress the biceps muscles more, while the overhand emphasizes the muscles of the back more.

When performing a chin-up, **don't**:

- Arch your back as you lift your body.
- Swing your legs or pull your knees up to help you reach the bar.
- Drop from the top position.

Do:

- Keep your abdominals tight.
- Perform all repetitions in a slow, controlled manner.
- Breathe, breathe, breathe.

Here's how you properly perform a chin-up:

1. Grab hold of the chin bar, with your hands several inches wider apart than shoulder width.

2. Keep your palms facing toward your body. Lift your feet off the floor and cross your ankles.

3. Pull your body to the heavens and touch your upper chest to the bar. (Most people try to inch their chin over the top. By focusing on your chest, you ensure that you really work your back.)

4. Pause briefly and return gradually (don't drop down) to the initial starting position, with your arms fully extended to get a good stretch.

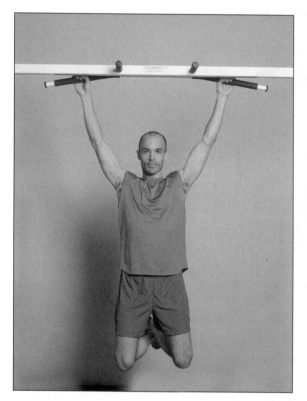 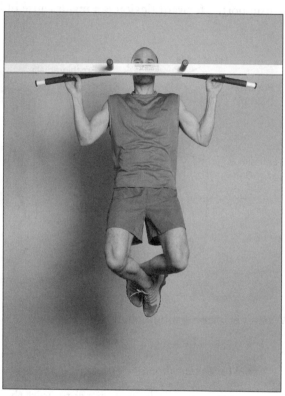

Chin-up start/finish position (left). Chin-up middle position (right).

Dumbbell Rows

Dumbbell rows emphasize the lats, middle traps, and rhomboids. The key to performing dumbbell rows is choosing a weight that allows you to squeeze the shoulder blade back on the positive phase of the movement, with control. If you have to jerk the dumbbell up with your body, you're not performing an effective set—and that means your muscles are not getting any stronger, no matter how much weight you're hoisting.

Another key to performing this exercise effectively without causing harm is to keep the leg on the side you're working on the floor. This lends support to your back as you're leaning forward. (Unsupported forward flexion is a major cause of lower-back pain.)

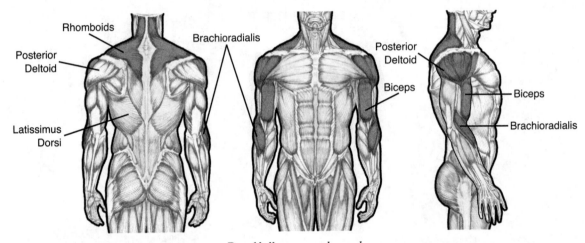

Dumbbell row: muscles used.

When performing a dumbbell row, **don't:**

- Arch your back.
- Move your shoulder excessively.
- Swing your body in an effort to hoist the weight.
- Twist your torso.

Do:

- Keep your abdominals tight and your back erect.
- Keep your shoulder and torso down and parallel to the floor.

Here's how you properly perform a dumbbell row:

1. Place your left hand and your left knee on a bench, and position your right foot on the floor at a comfortable distance from the bench.

2. Reach down with your right hand and grab the dumbbell.

3. Lift the dumbbell off the floor, keeping your right arm straight. Your right palm should be facing the bench.

4. Keeping your upper arm near your torso, slowly pull the dumbbell up to your right shoulder, as if you were sawing a piece of wood.

5. Pause briefly, and slowly return the dumbbell to the starting position.

6. Repeat with your left arm (with your right hand and right knee on the bench).

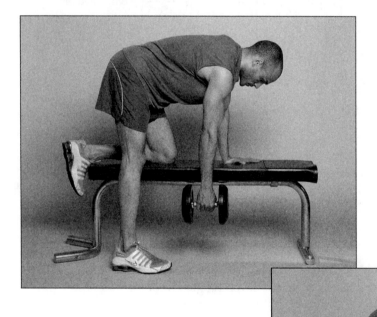

Dumbbell row start/finish position (top). Dumbbell row middle position (bottom).

Upright Rows

Many people think of the upright row as a shoulder exercise. It is a good way to work your deltoids and biceps, but it's also a great way to hit the top section of your trapezius. That's why we've included it in the back section.

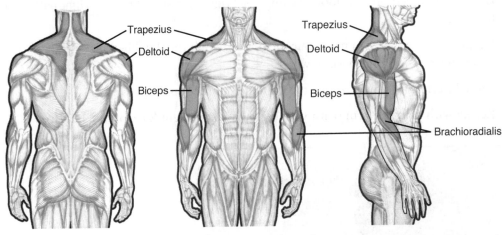

Upright rows: muscles used.

When performing an upright row, **don't:**

- Allow the bar to move away from your body while performing the repetition.
- Rock your body back and forth in an effort to lift the weight.

Do:

- Keep your abdominals tight and your back erect without leaning backward.
- Keep your elbows higher than your hands throughout the range of motion.

WEIGHT A MINUTE

People with shoulder impingement syndrome (a painful condition in which various structures are compressed in the shoulder joint when the arm is raised) should not perform this exercise.

Here's how you properly perform an upright row:

1. Stand with your feet shoulder width apart.

2. Hold the barbell slightly less than shoulder width apart, with your palms facing your thighs.

3. Pull up the bar until your hands are about level with your shoulders. Your elbows should be slightly higher than your hands.

4. Pause briefly and slowly return to the initial starting position.

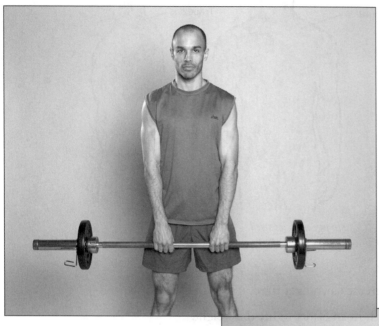

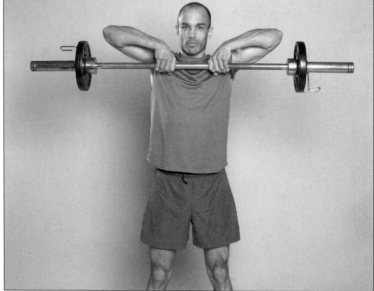

Upright row start/finish position (top). Upright row middle position (bottom).

Shrugs

While the upright row works your biceps and deltoids in addition to your trapezius, shrugs work the traps without involving those other muscles. Shrugs may look like a silly, insignificant exercise, but they're a great way to strengthen the traps. (To the uninitiated, someone doing shrugs looks terrifically undecided.) For anyone involved in contact sports or ones in which neck and head injuries are a possibility, shrugs can help you develop crucial stability.

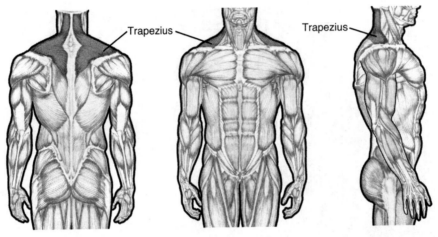

Shrug: muscles used.

When performing a shrug, **don't:**

- Let your range of motion decrease as you get tired.
- Rock your body back and forth in an effort to lift the weight.

Do:

- Keep your abdominal muscles tight and your back erect without leaning backward.
- Perform this exercise with a barbell for a change.

Here's how you properly perform a shrug:

1. Stand with your feet shoulder width apart.

2. Hold the dumbbells wider apart than shoulder width, with your palms facing your thighs.

3. Keeping your arms and legs straight, move the bar as high as possible by trying to touch your shoulders to your ears.

4. Pause briefly, and slowly return to the initial starting position.

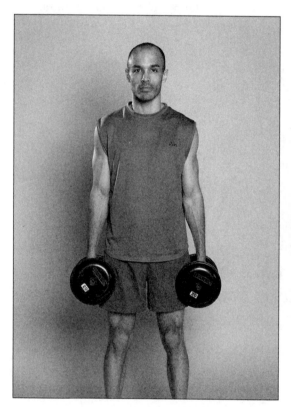 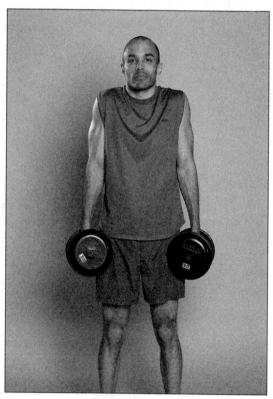

Shrug start/finish position (left). Shrug middle position (right).

Lat Time

Lat pull-downs are a standard part of virtually every lifter's routine. Done correctly, a lat pull-down will turn a blocky or narrow back into that much-sought-after V shape. Furthermore, if you're a swimmer, rock climber, rower, or any type of athlete who would benefit from a powerful upper body, this exercise is for you.

You can do two types of lat pull-downs: behind the neck or to the chest. With the behind-the-neck exercise, you might have a tendency to jut your neck forward, putting it in an awkward position, especially if you're using too much weight. For this reason, we prefer the chest variation because the neck is kept in a more stable position.

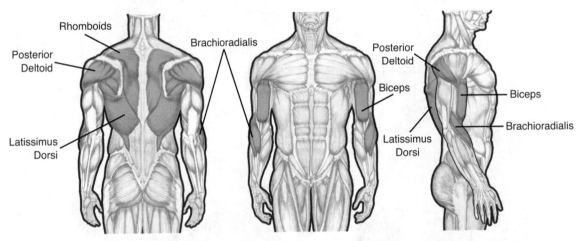

Lat pull-down: muscles used.

When performing a lat pull-down, **don't:**

- Come out of your seat on the way up.

- Swing your body back and forth in an effort to lift the weight.

- Slouch as you bring the weight down.

Do:

- Keep your abs tight and your back erect.

- Squeeze your shoulder blades together as you bring the weight down behind your neck.

- Control the weight throughout the range of motion.

WEIGHT A MINUTE

Don't do lat pull-downs if you have shoulder impingement syndrome. The exercise can aggravate the condition.

Here's how you properly perform a lat pull-down:

1. Grab the bar with your palms facing away from your body, slightly wider apart than shoulder width.

2. Sit on the seat with your knees under the pads. (Remember to adjust the pads if your knees don't fit snuggly yet comfortably.)

3. Lean back slightly.

4. Pull the bar to your collarbone.

5. Pause briefly and slowly return to the initial starting position.

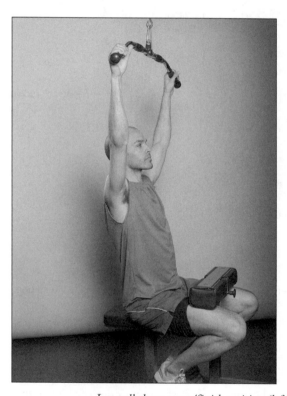 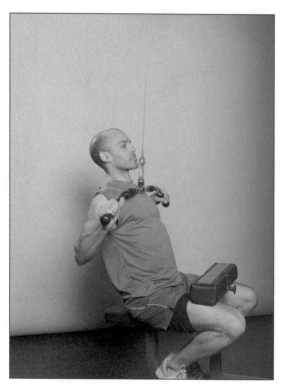

Lat pull-down start/finish position (left). Lat pull-down middle position (right).

Cable Rows

The cable row machine works the lats, middle traps, and rhomboids. Remember to keep your back erect even as you lean forward to return to the start position. As you pull the handle toward you—the initial pull is where your lats are worked—remember to keep your chest up and squeeze your shoulder blades together. (This is where the traps and rhomboids are worked.) As in virtually every exercise we recommend, perform cable rows slowly, exhaling on the positive phase of the movement (in this case, the pull toward the chest).

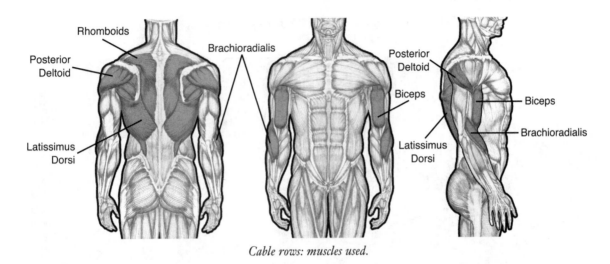

Cable rows: muscles used.

SPOT ME

Several different handles are available for this exercise. Experiment with them until you decide which one feels the most comfortable.

When performing a cable row, **don't:**

- Swing your upper body back and forth in an effort to lift the weight.
- Allow the weight stack being lifted to slam or bounce against the remainder of the weight stack between repetitions.
- Perform the exercise rapidly.
- Arch your back.

Do:

- Keep your abdominals tight and your back erect.
- Keep your knees slightly bent.
- Squeeze your shoulder blades together at the finish position.

Here's how you properly perform a cable row:

1. Sit down and place your feet against the foot platform.

2. Grab the bar and lean back slightly.

3. Pull the bar to your midsection.

4. Pause briefly and slowly return to the starting position, with your arms fully extended.

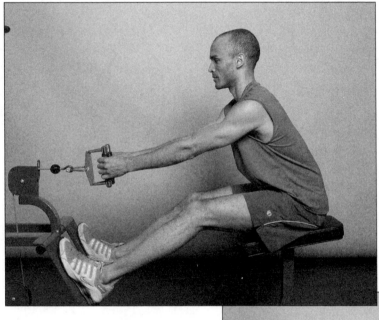

Cable row start/finish position (top). Cable row middle position (bottom).

Back Extension

Most of the exercises in this chapter focus on the muscles of your upper and middle back, but we've yet to get to the erector spinae muscles of your lower back. Strengthening those muscles is crucial in ensuring proper posture and preventing lower-back pain. Considering that the majority of people experience lower-back pain at some time in their lives, it's not a bad idea to do whatever's possible to decrease your chances of becoming a statistic. The 45° back extension bench is an effective and safe way to work those erector spinae.

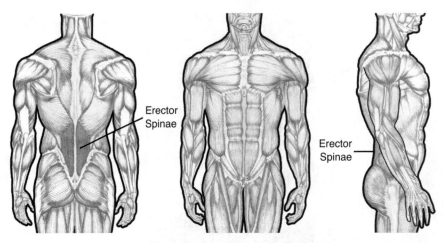

Back extension: muscles used.

When performing a back extension, **don't**:

- Push with your legs.
- Throw your head back.
- Swing back quickly.
- Hyperextend your back or neck.

Do:

- Keep your head in a neutral position.
- Control your weight in both directions.

Here's how you properly perform a back extension:

1. Be sure your heels are securely placed on the foot platform.

2. Begin by "folding" at the waist and letting your head hang down toward the floor.

3. Raise your torso until it's straight.

4. Pause at the fully extended position and slowly return to the starting position.

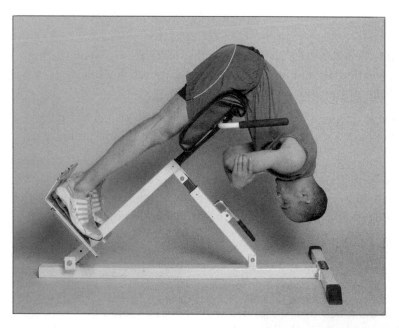

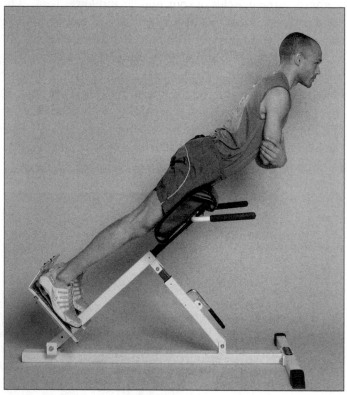

Back extension start/finish position (top). Back extension middle position (bottom).

Don't Do It

If you've read this far, you don't need to be a detective to figure out that we're fans of weightlifting. We like it for young and old, big and small, male and female. It's great for preventing injuries, improving sports performance, and helping you look good and feel better.

Still, lifting is not without some inherent dangers. Unfortunately, we see it all the time. Virtually every time we're in any gym—bare bones or high end—we see people doing exercises that make us cringe.

Throughout the next few chapters, as we introduce exercises that we like, we also occasionally highlight some of the most common and egregious mistakes we see in the weight room. After all, the only thing worse than a workout that doesn't help you get any stronger is one that injures you.

Here are a couple back exercises that we'd like to see you avoid.

Oh-No Bent Rows

Earlier in this chapter, we showed you dumbbell rows—a perfectly effective and safe way to strengthen the muscles of your middle and lower back. The only bad thing we can say about the dumbbell row is that you have to do the exercise with one arm at a time. Unfortunately, instead of using dumbbells for the exercise, many lifters use a barbell and take care of both sides of their body in one fell swoop. The problem is that while you're working out the muscles on both sides of your lower back, you're also compromising safety by bending forward. (In case you're brushing up for a biomechanics test, the technical term for this is unsupported forward flexion.) We're not suggesting that you'll get hurt any and every time you bend forward at the waist, but we do question the wisdom of doing it that way when there's a safer alternative. By placing your knee and nonworking hand on the bench during the dumbbell version, you protect your lower back yet still get every bit as good a workout for the muscles in your back.

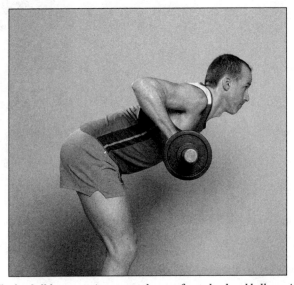

The barbell bent row is not nearly as safe as the dumbbell version.

Good Morning

While we're being picky about back exercises, let's look at the physical therapist's best friend—an exercise known as the good morning. In the good morning, you place a barbell across your back, bend forward at the waist, and then return to an upright, standing position. The idea of the good morning is to strengthen your lower back—just like back extensions do. It may do that, but it also jeopardizes the structures of your lower back in the process.

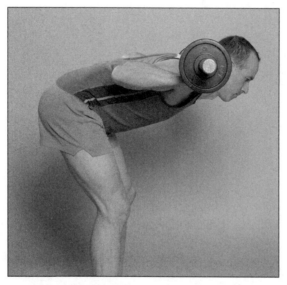

Skip the good mornings in favor of a safer alternative, like the back extension.

Chest or Bust

In This Chapter

- Deciding whether to bench or bust
- Knowing whether to go flat, incline, or decline
- Doing dips
- Learning chest machine options

Bulging arms and a chiseled chest may be the ideal for American men, but the bench press—one of the three powerlifting disciplines—is generally the signature lift men use to demonstrate how strong they are. Often you'll hear weightlifters ask each other, "What's your bench?" the way runners ask each other how fast they can run a 10K.

Oddly enough, the bench press, the exercise that builds the muscles in your chest, may be the most abused and overpopularized lift of them all. Why? A thick, sculpted chest is the body part men often assume will impress women. Because this lift has become such a benchmark of strength, too many men put too much weight on the bar too much of the time. The result often leads to shoulder injuries as well as bruised egos.

Pecs to Flex

The *pectoral* muscles (pecs) span the upper chest wall and are largely responsible for pushing and throwing movements. There are actually two pectoral muscles—the *pectoralis major* (the muscle we're concentrating on for weightlifting purposes) and the *pectoralis minor* (not shown), running beneath the pectoralis major from the third, fourth, and fifth ribs to the scapula (or shoulder blade); the pectoralis minor often gets extremely tight in people who have poor posture and needs to be massaged to get released.

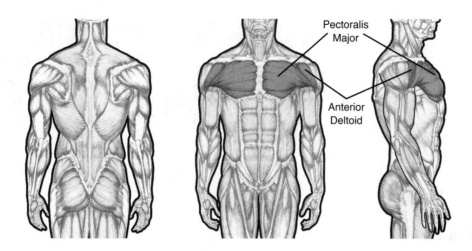

Why strong pecs? For the following reasons:

- If you play baseball or any other sport that involves throwing, strong pecs can give you that added *oomph*.

- If you're a swimmer, building your pecs will get you from one side of the pool to the other a bit quicker.

- If you're taking boxing classes or practicing the martial arts, strong pecs can make your punch a little harder.

Following are some basic exercises to get you started in the gym. Remember …

- Do them all slowly and under control—your muscles and joints will thank you.

- Breathe out as you push; breathe in as you return to the starting position.

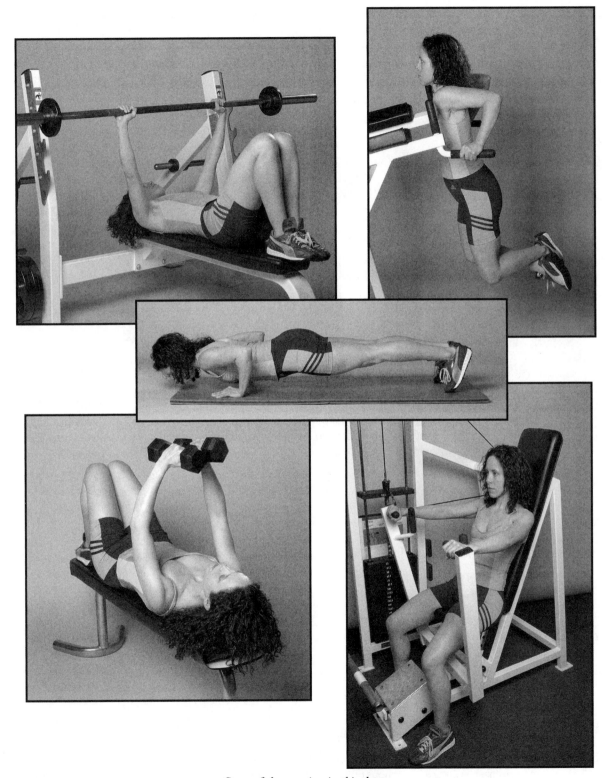

Some of the exercises in this chapter.

The Bench

The bench press, also known as the chest press, is a standard part of virtually every strength program. Its primary focus is the pectoralis major muscles, although it also works the front of the deltoid and the triceps. As we mentioned earlier, don't get caught up in the "How much can you lift?" game. Focus on form, and the strength gains will take care of themselves.

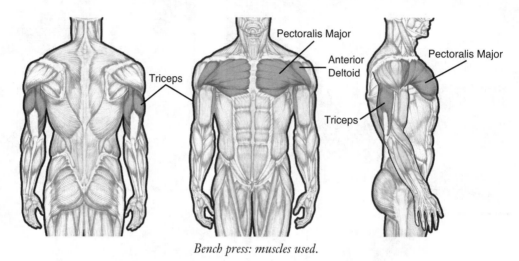

Bench press: muscles used.

FLEX FACTS

The bench press is significantly different for powerlifters than for noncompetitive athletes. In competition, powerlifters arch their backs, dig their feet into the floor, and grind their shoulder blades into the bench. This anchoring gives them enough leverage to drive the bar up off their chest to successfully make their one-repetition max.

When performing a bench press, **don't**:

- Arch your back.
- Lift your buttocks off the bench.
- Move your legs or feet—keep them stationary for better support.
- Snap or lock your elbows at the end position.
- Bounce the barbell off your chest.
- Hold your breath.

Do:

- Keep your abdomen tight and your back flat.
- Use a firm but relaxed grip.

WEIGHT A MINUTE

The temptation to try a maximal lift on a bench press (or any other lift) is one we urge you to ignore. One-rep maximal lifts place an enormous orthopedic stress on your body and tend to shoot your blood pressure through the roof—and they're not the best way to get stronger. Leave maximal lifts to competitive lifters.

Here's how you properly perform a bench press:

1. Lie on your back with your feet either flat on the floor or, if your feet don't touch the floor, without your back arching.

2. Bend your knees and put your feet on the bench. (When you put your feet on the bench, you reduce the potential stress on your back and isolate the muscles a bit more. It also means you use less weight.) In either case, keep your back flat.

3. Grab the bar with a grip slightly wider apart than shoulder width.

4. Lift the bar from the uprights, or have a spotter assist you.

5. Slowly lower the bar to your chest, stopping at the highest part of your chest (at the nipple line); then return to the initial starting position.

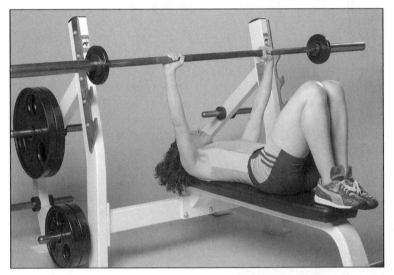

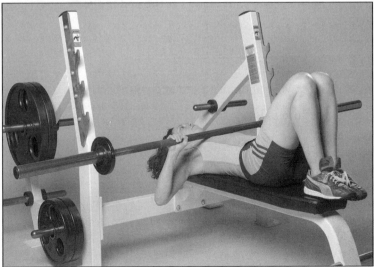

Bench press start/finish position (top). Bench press middle position (bottom).

Goin' Uphill

The incline bench press works on the upper part of your pecs. Bodybuilders tend to focus on defining every single muscle possible, so they perform flat, incline, and decline bench presses to bring out their pecs as much as they can.

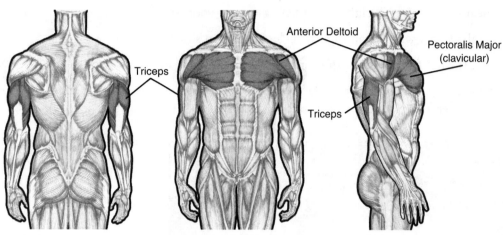

Incline press: muscles used.

When performing an incline press, **don't:**

- Lift your buttocks off the bench.
- Arch your back.
- Move your legs or your feet.
- Bounce the barbell off your chest.
- Snap or lock your elbows at the end range.
- Hold your breath.

Do:

- Keep your abdomen tight and your back flat.
- Be sure to lower the bar to just below your collarbone.

Here's how you properly perform an incline press:

1. Lie on the bench and place your feet either flat on the floor or on the footrest (if one is present).

2. Grab the bar with a grip slightly wider apart than shoulder width.

3. Lift the bar from the uprights, or have a spotter assist you.

4. Slowly lower the bar until it touches the upper part of your chest, just below your collarbone; then slowly return to the initial starting position.

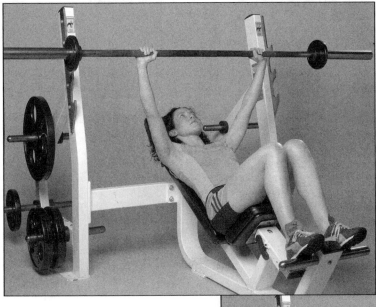

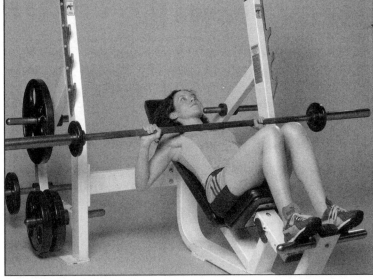

Incline press start/finish position (top). Incline press middle position (bottom).

Down We Go

The decline bench is the kissin' cousin of the incline variety because it works the lower part of your chest. Essentially, you follow the same procedure as the flat and incline bench. The tricky part is sliding under the bar without smacking your head.

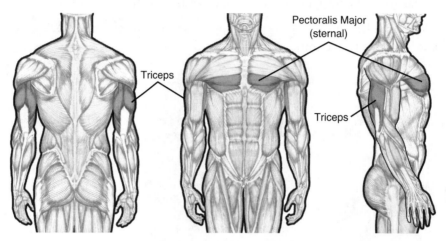

Decline press: muscles used.

When performing a decline press, **don't:**

- Lock your elbows as you straighten your arms.
- Bounce the bar off your chest.
- Arch your back.
- Hold the bar with a *suicide grip!*

> **DEFINITION**
>
> The **suicide grip** (or thumbless grip) refers to gripping the barbell with your thumb on the same side of the barbell as your four other fingers. Some lifters find this more comfortable, but it is extremely dangerous because the bar could slip from your hands. We don't recommend it.

Do:

- Keep your abdominals tight.
- Keep your head on the bench.
- Lower the bar to your nipple line.

Here's how you properly perform a decline press:

1. Lie on the bench, putting your feet under the support provided.

2. Grab the bar with a grip slightly wider apart than shoulder width.

3. Lift from the uprights, or have a spotter assist you.

4. Slowly lower the bar to your chest just below the nipple line; then return to the initial starting position.

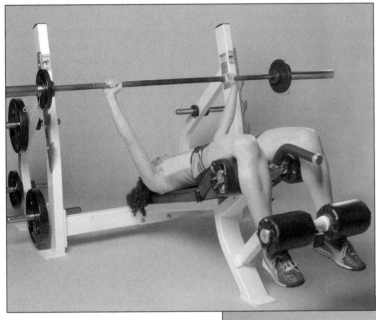

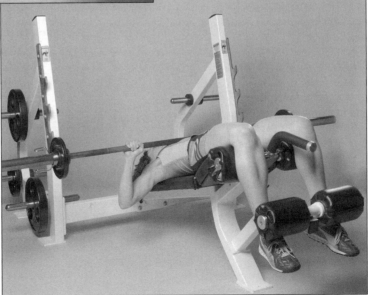

Decline press start/finish position (top). Decline press middle position (bottom).

Dips

Most people find dips extremely difficult, with good reason—they are. They also happen to be one of the best exercises for your chest and upper body that money can buy. If you can't do even one, don't despair. Nowadays, most well-equipped gyms have an assisted dip machine or Gravitron that helps you by pushing up as you stand on a platform. Better to use the help than to use bad form with your full body weight.

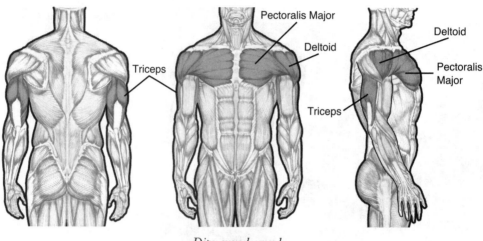

Dips: muscles used.

When performing a dip, **don't:**

- Snap or lock your elbows as you push yourself up.

- Arch your back.

- Allow your elbows to jut out toward the side; keep them pointed directly backward.

Do:

- Keep your chest up.

- Keep your chin tucked and your eyes focused on an object directly in front of you.

- Keep your knees bent.

Here's how you properly perform a dip:

1. Stand between the two handles, bend your knees, and hold yourself up by keeping your elbows straight. If you're using an assisted dip machine, keep your feet flat on the platform.

2. Slowly bend your elbows, lowering your body as far as you can comfortably—ideally, until your upper arms are parallel to the floor; then return to the initial starting position with a smooth, outward breath.

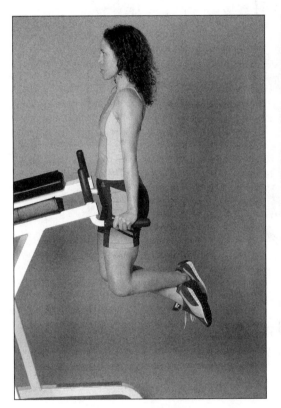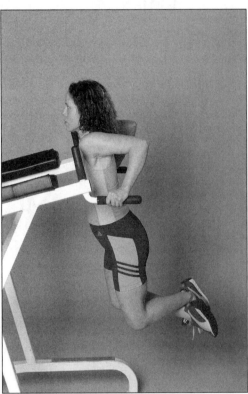

Dip start/finish position (left). Dip middle position (right).

Push, Please

The push-up is perhaps the most classic of all strength-training exercises. Think back to grade school when you did that first facsimile of what Marines and Navy SEALs do more of than any other exercise. While the push-up is as common as a pigeon in New York City, it is an important exercise to incorporate into your regimen, especially considering the fact that you can do it anywhere, any time.

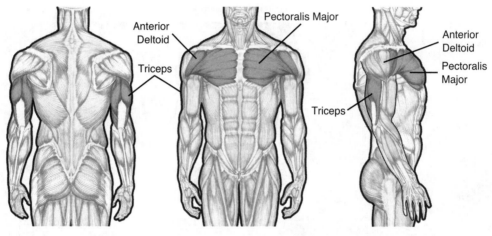

Push-ups: muscles used.

When performing a push-up, **don't:**

- Allow your back to sag while assuming the up position.
- Snap or lock your elbows while at the end position.
- Rest between the start position and the end position.

Do:

- Keep your abdomen tight.
- Keep your head facing the floor without arching your neck.

Here's how you properly perform a push-up:

1. Lie on the floor with your legs together and your hands on the floor pointing forward and just outside your shoulders.

2. Keep your back and legs straight.

3. Slowly push your body from the floor until your elbows are straight, then slowly return to the initial starting position. Concentrate on keeping your back straight and your rhythm even.

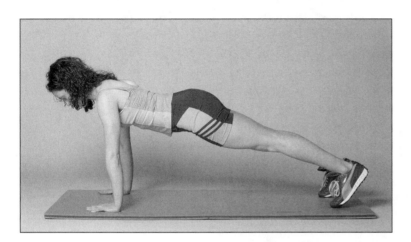

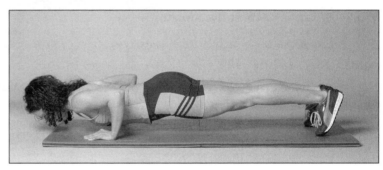

Push-up start/finish position (top). Push-up middle position (bottom).

Flying Solo

Dumbbell flyes are an extremely challenging exercise for your chest because they emphasize the pec major without assistance from the anterior delts and the triceps. It's important to concentrate on your form and keep a smooth and continuous flow to this exercise. Any herky-jerkiness will likely result in injury. If you find yourself cheating, use less weight.

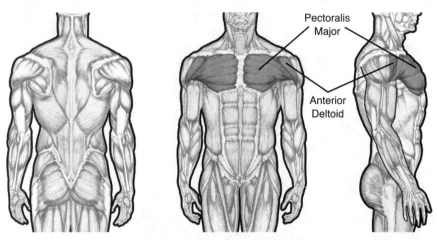

Chest flyes: muscles used.

When performing a chest flye, **don't:**

- Use too much weight with this exercise. You can cause serious injury to your *rotator cuff* muscles in your shoulder.

- Straighten your elbows—you can put excessive stress on the joint.

- Arch your back.

Do:

- Get a good stretch at the start position.

- Focus on form.

Here's how you properly perform a chest flye:

1. Lie on the bench either with your feet flat on the floor or with your knees bent and your feet on the bench.

2. Stretch out your arms, with one dumbbell in each hand.

3. Slightly bend your elbows.

4. Slowly bring your arms together until the dumbbells almost touch; then return to the initial starting position. Picture the wings of a soaring bird, and you've got the right idea.

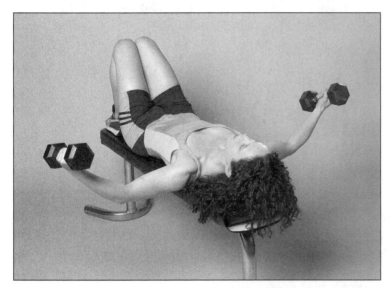

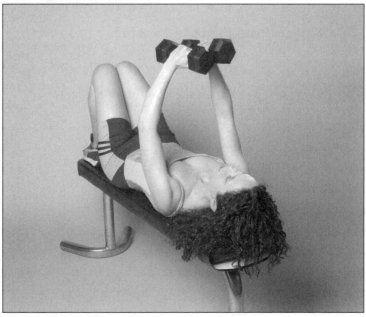

Chest flye start/finish position (top). Chest flye middle position (bottom).

Chest Press

This machine is the rough equivalent of the flat bench press. Some machines place you flat on your back; others put you in a seated position. In either case, the machine works the same primary muscles as the bench press but recruits fewer stabilizers because it keeps you in a fixed plane.

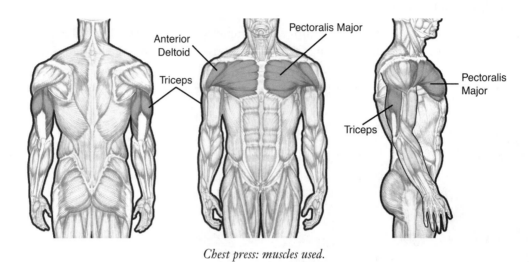

Chest press: muscles used.

When performing a chest press, **don't:**

- Snap or lock your elbows as you press forward.

- Arch your back.

- Lift your upper body or head from the back pad.

- Lift your buttocks from the seat pad.

Do:

- Keep your feet flat on the floor or on the footrest.

- Keep your abdomen tight.

Here's how you properly perform a chest press:

1. Position yourself on the machine.

2. Keep your feet flat on the floor or on the footrest, if you have one to use. Remember, posture counts.

3. Place your hands on the handles.

4. Push the handles forward, focusing your attention on your pecs.

5. Finish the forward push just short of full extension; then slowly return to the starting position without relaxing completely.

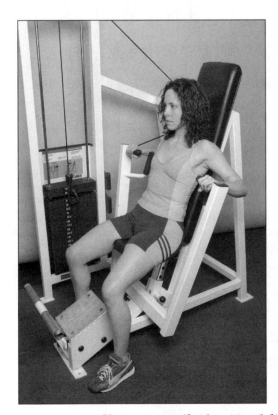 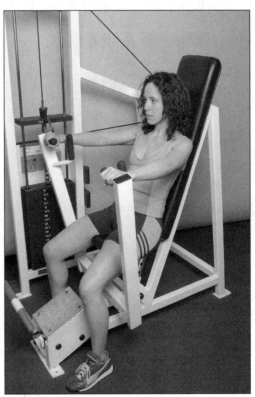

Chest press start/finish position (left). Chest press middle position (right).

Flye Machine

The flye machine (sometimes called a peck deck) is a terrific machine for isolating the pec muscles. It's analogous to the dumbbell flyes and enables you to isolate your pecs without using the muscles in your arms.

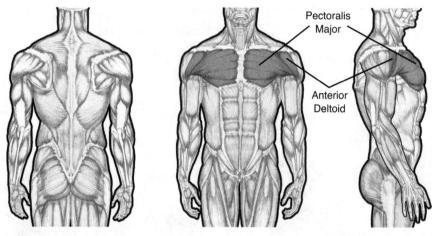

Pec deck: muscles used.

SPOT ME

The pec deck is the machine version of the flye, but in some ways, we actually prefer it. Both exercises isolate your pecs and eliminate your arm muscles, but the pec deck enables you to work through a broader range of motion and keeps constant pressure on the muscle.

When performing a pec deck, **don't**:

- Lift your elbows off the arm pads.
- Lift your upper body or head from the back pad.
- Lift your buttocks from the seat pad.
- Slam the stack weights between repetitions.
- Arch your back.

Do:

- Keep your feet flat on the floor or on the footrest.
- Keep your abdomen tight.

If you have a shoulder impingement, refrain from doing this exercise.

Here's how you properly perform a pec deck:

1. Position yourself on the machine.

2. Keep your feet flat on the floor or on the footrest.

3. Place your forearms on either side of the pads.

4. Without moving your upper body or lifting your head from the back pad, bring your elbows as close together as possible by pushing against the arm pads.

5. Resist the temptation to twist, squirm, or otherwise recruit any other body parts. Remember that the focus is on form and elegance.

6. Return to the initial starting position.

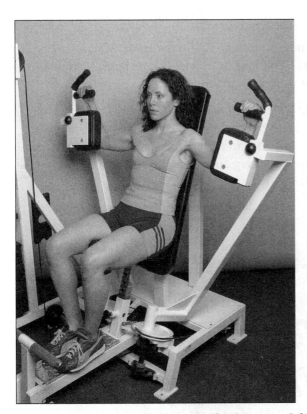 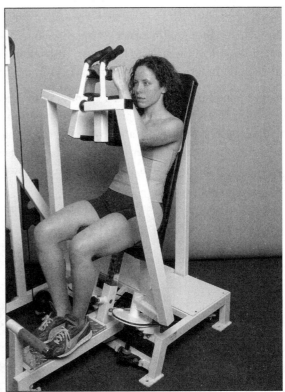

Pec deck start/finish position (left). Pec deck middle position (right).

Don't Do It

Since Chapter 1, we've been stressing that the goal of lifting should be to *gain* strength, not to *demonstrate* strength, yet many lifters persist in the dangerous and counterproductive practice of "maxing out" on the bench press. Worse still, the form they use to help show off their "strength" generally ranges from poor to atrocious.

Here are the most common mistakes we see:

- Arching the back
- Holding the breath
- Lowering the bar too fast
- Bouncing the bar off the chest

Sure, this makes it a lot easier to impress your friends, but all too often, the result of bad bench press form is a shoulder, wrist, or back injury. These form faux pas keep Deidre's physical therapy practice thriving but don't do much for the lifters who commit them.

Proper bench press form means keeping your knees bent and your feet flat on the floor at all times. If your back arches off the bench in this position, place your feet on the bench or use 45-pound plates as risers. Slowly lift and lower the bar. Hold 3 seconds in each direction and pause for a split-second at your chest; never bounce the bar. Exhale on the way up and inhale on the way down. Last but not least, always use a spotter. If one isn't available, use a machine or dumbbells.

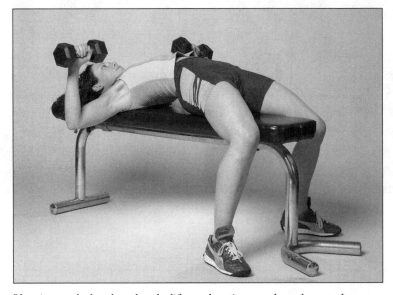

Cheating on the bench makes the lift much easier—and much more dangerous.

The Shoulders

In This Chapter

- Learning the anatomy of a shoulder
- Performing delts exercises

Atlas carried the world on his shoulders. Often you hear people say, "That must be a load off your shoulders!" or "You've been shouldering a huge burden the last few weeks." In other words, the shoulders are known to bear the brunt of hard work and mental stress. While most people relish training their chest, arms, back, and even their legs, the shoulders are one of the most neglected body parts.

Why? The shoulders (the *deltoids*, or delts) are the muscles located at the top of your arm. This muscle actually has three parts: the *anterior deltoid*, which raises the arm from the front; the *medial deltoid*, which raises the arm from the side; and the *posterior deltoid*, which draws the arm backward. Together these muscles form a triangle on your shoulder (hence the name *deltoid*, as in the Greek *delta*). These muscles are amazingly versatile but relatively small, and therefore fatigue easily. When you start training your shoulders, you're likely to notice, first, how weak they are, and, second, how quickly they respond if you train them diligently.

DEFINITION

The **deltoid** is divided into three sections—the **anterior deltoid** is the front section, the **medial deltoid** is in the middle, and the **posterior deltoid** is at the back.

Another seldom-considered set of muscles plays a large role in the health and welfare of your shoulders: the rotator cuff. The rotator cuff muscles are located beneath the deltoids, and their function is to keep your long arm bone (the *humerus*) from slipping out of joint. Compared to the deltoids, these muscles are small and seldom thought about—until an injury occurs, often while straining under the load of too much weight on the bench press.

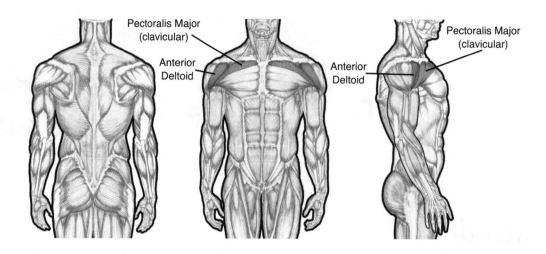

Not sure how your rotator cuff functions? Try this: stick out your arm to the side, with your elbow locked. Now twist your arm from side to side. Which muscle gets the job done? The loyal rotator cuff. The supraspinatus also assists your deltoids in initiating the outward movement of your arm from the side. And it provides stability to the joint when you throw a ball, Frisbee, javelin—you get the picture. Having said all that, it should come as no surprise to hear that a thorough shoulder workout encompasses the deltoids and the rotator cuff muscles as well.

FLEX FACTS

Anatomy students always remember the muscles of the rotator cuff with the acronym SITS. The rotator cuff consists of four muscles—supraspinatus, infraspinatus, teres minor, and subscapularis.

Should I?

Why strong shoulders? If you play racquet sports or baseball, or want to be the next Tom Brady, improving your shoulder strength is a must. (The shoulders will help you in throwing the football and couldn't hurt in your quest to find a Brazilian supermodel wife.) From a cosmetic point of view, powerfully built shoulders give your upper body more width. Add buff shoulders to a sculpted back, and your waist will look significantly smaller. (And women, take notice: train your shoulders long enough, and you won't need to use those shoulder pads in your clothes.)

Laying down a good foundation when you begin to work on your deltoids is extremely important. The last thing you need to worry about is the amount of weight you're using. Always be sure that your form is excellent and that you're not using your whole body to initiate the exercise.

When working your shoulders, it's important to maintain good form and posture and to move the weight in a smooth, controlled manner.

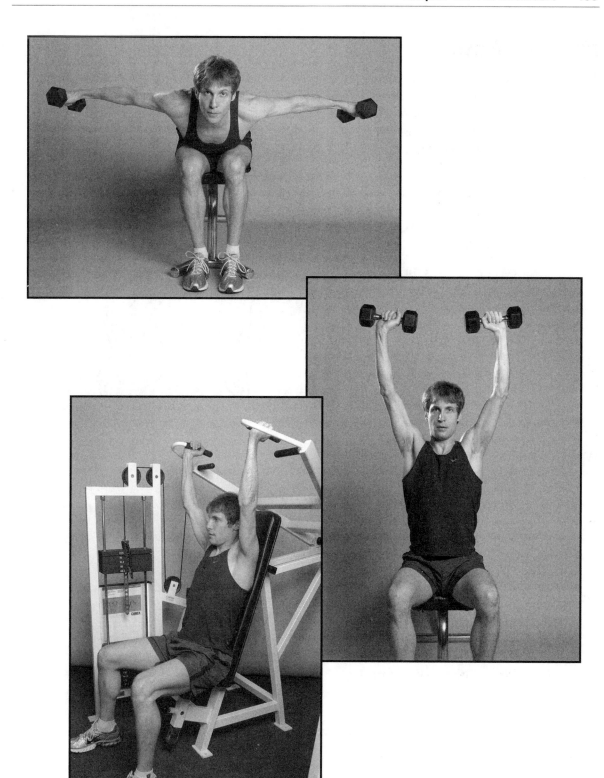

Some of the exercises in this chapter.

Military Action

The military press is a great basic compound exercise to do. It works not only the deltoids, but also the triceps, and can be done in both sitting and standing positions. Deidre prefers to perform it while standing because it's easier to control the position of the lower back, especially with heavier weights. No matter which position you choose, keep your back erect, your abdominals tight, and your head in neutral position. If it sounds like we're sticklers for form, that's because we are.

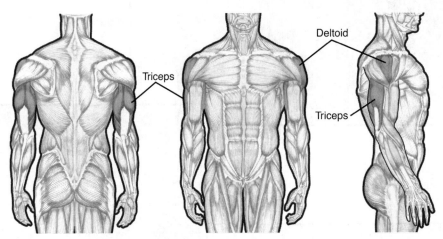

Military press: muscles used.

When performing a military press, **don't:**

- Arch your back.
- Clang the dumbbells together.
- Allow your elbows to dip below the start position.
- Twist from your waist to nudge the weight upward.

Do:

- Keep your abs tight.
- Keep your head and neck straight.
- Pay strict attention to your form.

Here's how you properly perform a military press:

1. Sit with your feet on the foot platform, if there is one, with a dumbbell in each hand.

2. Bring up the dumbbells with your palms facing forward.

3. Hold them like a driver signaling to make a right turn—in a position of 90° of shoulder abduction and 90° of elbow flexion.

4. Slowly straighten your arms overhead, finishing with a slight bend in your elbows.

5. While maintaining control of the weight, return to the initial starting position.

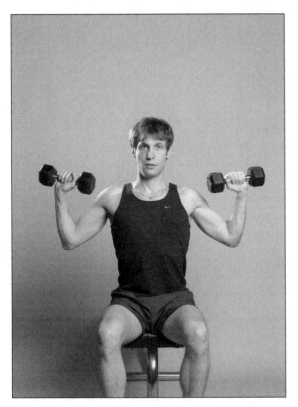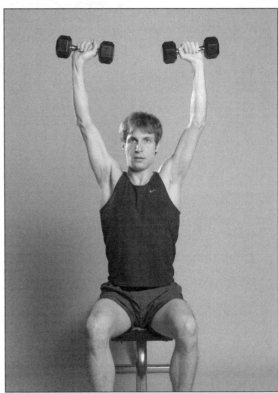

Military press start/finish position (left). Military press middle position (right).

Lateral Raises

Lateral raises are a great exercise for isolating the middle deltoids. (They are considered one-joint exercises because the only joint flexing and extending is the shoulder joint. Military presses are two-joint exercises because two joints flex and extend.) Note that you use much lighter weight with lateral raises than with the military press. Also note that you need to keep your elbows slightly bent to take excess pressure off of them.

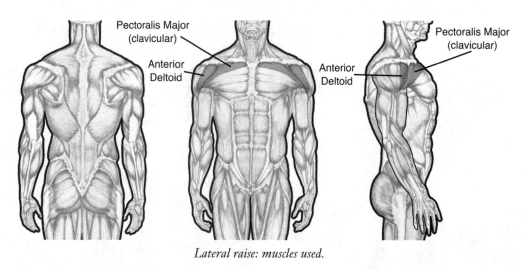

Lateral raise: muscles used.

When performing a lateral raise, **don't:**

- Raise your arms much above the parallel position.
- Dip your body downward as you lift the weights.
- Lean forward.
- Relax completely between repetitions.

Do:

- Keep your abdominals tight.
- Keep your weight evenly distributed on your feet.
- Maintain good posture.

Here's how you properly perform a lateral raise:

1. Sit at the end of a bench with your legs together.

2. Hold a dumbbell in each hand at your side, with your palms facing your legs.

3. With a slight bend in your elbows, raise the dumbbells away from the sides of your body until your arms are parallel to the floor.

4. Return to the starting position under control.

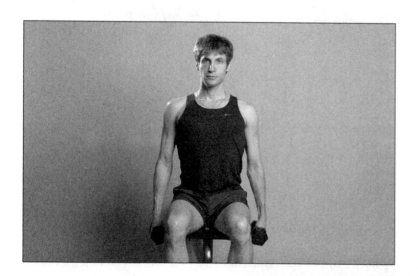

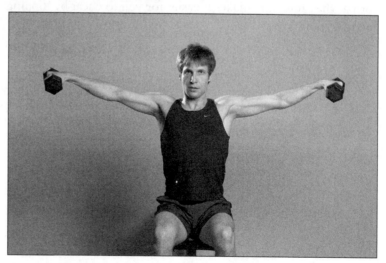

Lateral raise start/finish position (top). Lateral raise middle position (bottom).

Front Raises

If you're wondering why we're listing so many exercises for the shoulder, keep in mind that it is a three-part muscle and that you must work each muscle to get stronger as a whole. Front raises are another one-joint exercise, meaning that they isolate the anterior deltoid, which is the muscle you use to reach up to grab an apple off a tree.

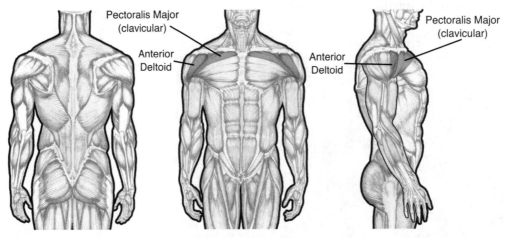

Front raise: muscles used.

Although you will see people exercising both arms at the same time, we prefer that you don't. Doing both at the same time makes it easier for you to cheat by dipping your body or arching your back as you raise both arms.

SPOT ME

Although we have shown the front raise exercise with palms facing downward, people who have shoulder impingement syndrome should not perform it in this fashion because it can worsen the condition. Instead, begin with your palms facing inward, and keep them facing inward throughout the exercise.

When performing a front raise, **don't**:

- Rock your body back and forth.

- Raise your arms above the parallel position.

Do:

- Keep your abs tight.

- Maintain good posture.

Here's how you properly perform a front raise:

1. Stand with your feet shoulder width apart and your knees slightly bent.

2. Hold a dumbbell in each hand at your sides, with your palms facing your legs.

3. Slowly raise one dumbbell in front of your body until your arm is parallel to the floor.

4. Slowly return to the starting position.

5. Do a complete set with one arm before beginning the next arm.

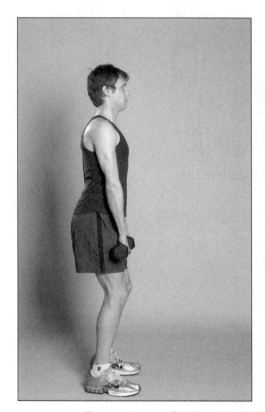 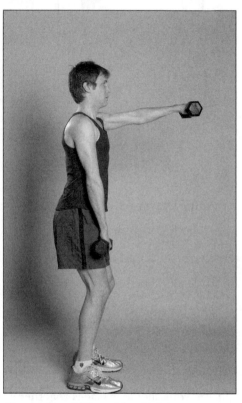

Front raise start/finish position (left). Front raise middle position (right).

Reverse Flyes

Reverse flyes are another one-joint exercise that isolates the posterior deltoid. For the whole muscle to get strong, you must work all its parts.

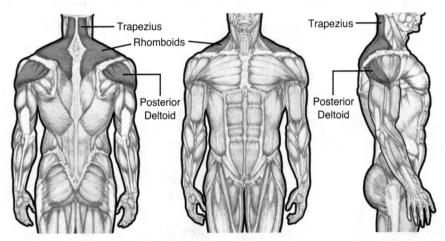

Reverse flyes: muscles used.

When performing a reverse flye, **don't:**

- Turn your head left or right.
- Raise your arms quickly, forcing your body forward.
- Allow the dumbbells to clang together.

Do:

- Keep your abs tight.
- Maintain slow, controlled movement throughout the exercise.
- Squeeze your shoulder blades together at the top of the movement.

Here's how you properly perform a reverse flye:

1. Sit on a flat bench and bend forward at your waist.

2. Let the dumbbells hang down at your sides.

3. Bend your elbows slightly as you raise the dumbbells away from your body.

4. Focus on squeezing your shoulder blades together.

5. With control, return to the starting position.

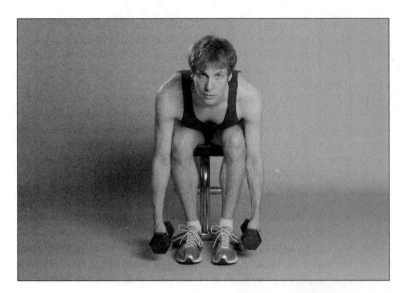

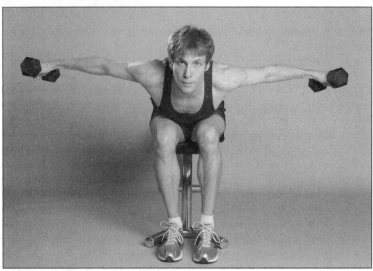

Reverse flye start/finish position (top). Reverse flye middle position (bottom).

Shoulder Press Machine

This machine is the kissin' cousin of the military press; however, unlike the free weight version, which requires copious amounts of concentration, using the shoulder press machine is safer (and easier) because you neither have to stabilize the weight nor worry about it falling against your will. That's also the reason we generally prefer the free weight version, but it's good to know this one as well.

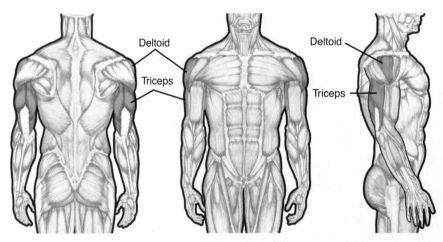

Shoulder press: muscles used.

 WEIGHT A MINUTE

People with lower back pain or shoulder impingement syndrome should not do this exercise.

When performing a shoulder press, **don't:**

- Lean backward.
- Lift your buttocks off the bench.
- Allow your elbows to snap or lock in the middle position.
- Allow the weight stack you're lifting to slam against the remaining weight stack between repetitions.

Do:

- Keep your abdominals tight and your back erect.
- Keep your head straight.

Here's how you properly perform a shoulder press:

1. Sit on the bench with your feet shoulder width apart.

2. Grasp the handles slightly wider than shoulder width apart.

3. Sit up straight and start your engine.

4. Push up the handles until your arms are just short of full extension.

5. Return to a position just short of the initial starting position, to keep tension on your muscles. Remember to maintain control of the downward part of the lift.

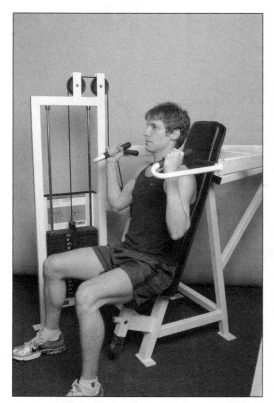 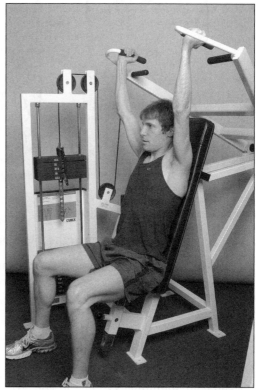

Shoulder press machine start/finish position (left). Shoulder press machine middle position (right).

Lateral Raise Machine

This machine virtually duplicates the free weight version of the lateral raise. Some people prefer using a machine because it requires less concentration; others like using free weights because it may be more comfortable for them and they maintain a bit more control. Try both, and you can make the call.

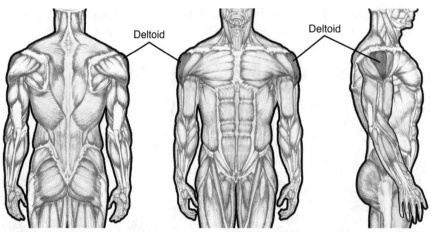

Deltoid   Deltoid

Lateral raise: muscles used.

When performing a lateral raise, **don't:**

- Lift your arms to a position higher than parallel.

- Allow the weight stack you're lifting to slam against the remaining weight stack between repetitions.

Do:

- Keep your upper body and head against the back pad to reduce the strain on your neck and back.

- Keep your abdominals tight and your back erect.

Here's how you properly perform a lateral raise:

1. Sit on the seat.

2. Position your upper arms against the arm pads, and lay your upper body against the back pad. Extend your elbows straight down, and bend your elbows to 90°, with your palms facing in.

3. Keep your arms fairly straight and raise them away from your body until they are parallel to the floor.

4. Return the weight gradually to a position just short of the initial starting position.

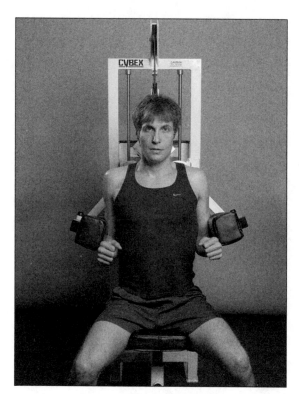 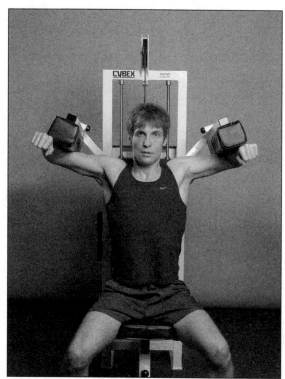

Lateral raise machine start/finish position (left). Lateral raise machine middle position (right).

The Arms

In This Chapter

- Building your biceps
- Boosting your triceps
- Working your wrists

Picture this: you walk into a gym for your first workout, and you're looking for a trainer. You see two trainers discussing amino acids by the office. Both have pleasing physiques, but one has huge arms. Which one do you want for your trainer? (Be honest.) Our practical experience says you go with Bobby Biceps.

Chew on this amusing "looks can be deceiving" tale: Jonathan used to work with a nutritionist who had implausibly muscular arms. Whenever they were together at the gym, people approached him with questions about arm exercises, despite the fact that he had no real exercise background. Jonathan, a lean endurance athlete (okay, a pencil neck) who had a Master's degree in exercise physiology, knew far more arm exercises than there are amino acids. Conversely, when people had questions pertaining to diet and losing weight, they came to Jonathan, assuming that he was the man to ask, even though Mr. Biceps had a Ph.D. in nutrition. Go figure.

Joe's Uncle Harry, a short, jovial guy who worked for years as a paper salesman, had biceps like cannonballs from lifting stacks of paper all day. Whenever he visited, Joe insisted that he make a muscle for Joe to squeeze. Even though he was only 5 feet, 5 inches, those prodigious pythons on Harry's upper arms made him feel large. The point is that bulging biceps have long been symbols of masculine strength. Perhaps the biggest reason for this is their highly visible location. Another reason they're so identified with strength is that often very strong men have very large arms.

Of course, a lot of this has to do with who you picked as your parents (in other words, genetics). Regardless, big or not so big, there are lots of real-life reasons to have strong biceps.

Bulging Biceps

The biceps span the front of the upper arm, beginning at the upper part of the long bone of your arm *(humerus)* and ending at the point just beyond where your elbow bends. The action of the biceps is to bend the elbow and to turn your palm up toward the ceiling. This action of flexion and supination is the way you show off when you make a muscle like Joe's lovable Uncle Harry.

Why strong biceps? For the following reasons:

- Assistance with exercises for larger body parts. If your biceps are weak, they won't be of much help when performing exercises for your back.

- Activities of daily living. If your biceps are weak, your arms will tire while carrying your kid from the car to the bedroom, carrying packages, or using a screwdriver.

- They look good. Right or wrong, big biceps are seen as a sign of strength.

Here's the skinny when it comes to your biceps: these smallish muscles are involved in virtually every pulling movement you do in the gym (lat pull-downs, cable rows, and many more). As a result, you don't have to do many concentrated biceps exercises. We also recommend that you save your biceps routine for one of the last groups of exercises you do. Why? If you exhaust your biceps first, you won't get an effective workout for your larger body parts because your biceps won't be able to withstand much more fatigue. So although they're good "show muscles," we don't want you to get carried away working your biceps.

When doing your arm exercises, pay careful attention to your technique and posture. That means sitting and standing in an erect yet relaxed position and lifting the weight slowly through a full range of motion.

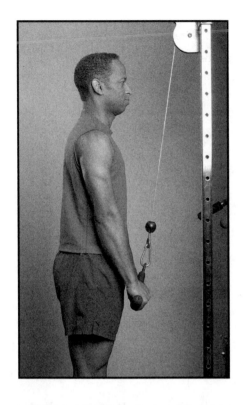

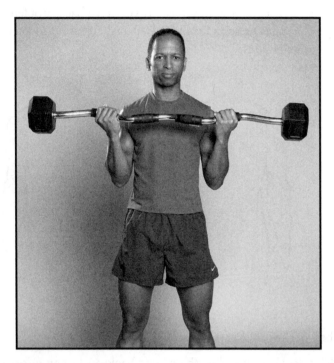

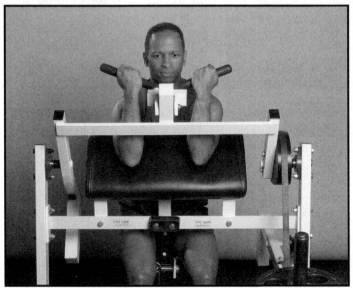

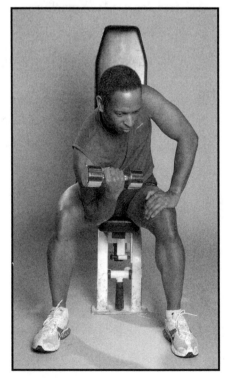

Some of the exercises in this chapter.

Standing Curls

This is the classic biceps exercise. If you have back problems, do this while standing against a wall. Even if you have a sound back, pay special attention to keeping your back straight and your elbows close to your sides.

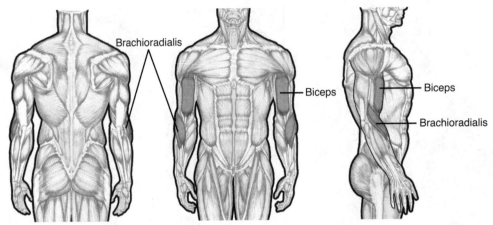

Standing curl: muscles used.

When performing a standing curl, **don't:**

- Rock back and forth or bend backward in an effort to get the weight up. If you must do this, you've used too much weight and should lighten the load.

- Let your elbows wander up as you lift.

- Curl the weight all the way up to your shoulders.

Do:

- Keep your knees slightly bent and your abdomen held tight; this protects your back.

- Keep your elbows tucked in close to your body.

Here's how you properly perform a standing curl:

1. Grip the barbell with your palms facing outward, shoulder width apart.

2. Stand with your feet approximately shoulder width apart.

3. Begin with the bar resting on the front of your thighs.

4. Slowly raise the bar by bending your elbows toward your shoulders; slowly lower the bar to the front of your thighs.

5. Control the downward motion during this negative phase.

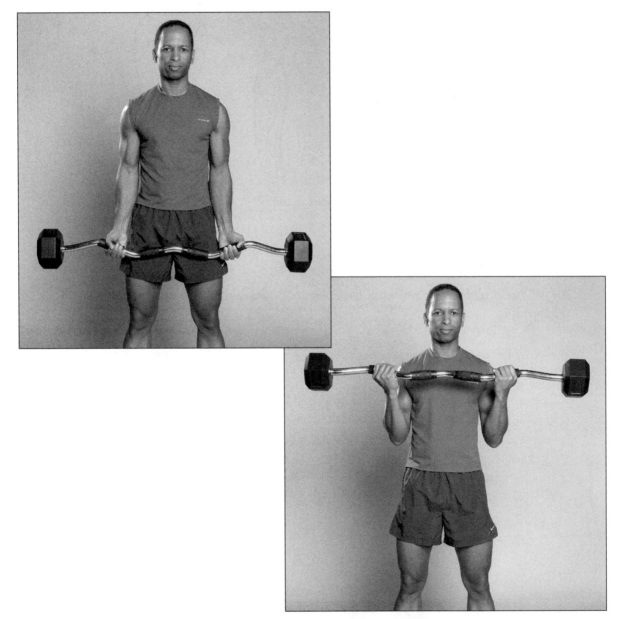

Standing curl start/finish position (top). Standing curl middle position (bottom).

Dumbbell Curls

Dumbbell curls are similar to barbell curls, except that, well, you're using dumbbells and, instead of working both biceps at the same time, you have the option of lifting them simultaneously or alternately. Because alternating gives the muscle time to rest as the other arm is working, we prefer to work both arms together.

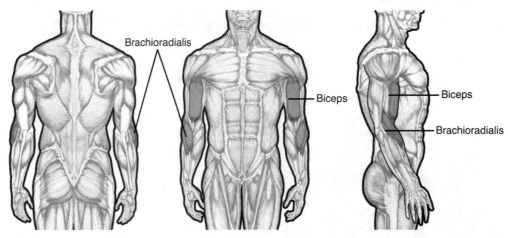

Dumbbell curl: muscles used.

When performing a dumbbell curl, **don't:**

- Shrug your shoulders as you raise the dumbbells.
- Rock back and forth or arch your back. Again, decrease the weight if you find this happening.

Do:

- Keep your elbows pinned in close to your body.
- Keep your knees slightly bent if standing, and keep your abdomen tight, whether you are standing or sitting, to protect your back.

Here's how you properly perform a dumbbell curl:

1. Stand (or sit) with a dumbbell in each hand, with your palms facing inward.

2. Slowly bend your elbow. As you do, begin to twist your wrists so your palms are facing upward.

3. Stop just short of your shoulders.

4. Slowly straighten your elbow. As you do, begin to twist your wrists so your palms are facing inward again.

5. Return to your initial starting position.

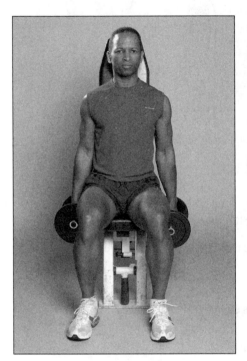 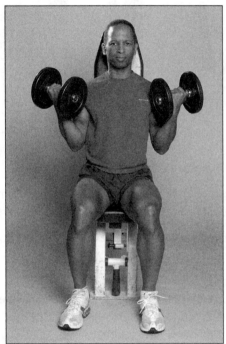

Dumbbell curl start/finish position (left). Dumbbell curl middle position (right).

Concentration Curls

Concentration curls are a great way to ensure that you use strict form on your curls. Because they're a little harder, you'll have to use less weight than in the previous exercise.

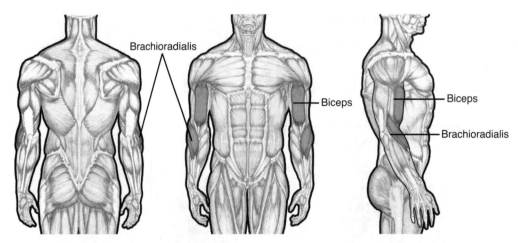

Concentration curls: muscles used.

When performing a concentration curl, **don't:**

- Lean or rock backward and forward in an effort to hoist the dumbbell—you could hurt your back. If your form isn't perfect, immediately lessen the weight.

- Move your leg from side to side in an effort to help you lift the weight.

Do:

- Keep your abdomen tight and your back erect as you are leaning forward.

Here's how you properly perform a concentration curl:

1. With a dumbbell in your hand, sit on a bench, lean forward, and rest your arm on the inner part of your thigh.

2. Keep your palm facing your opposite thigh.

3. Raise the dumbbell by slowly bending to a point just short of your shoulder.

4. Lower the dumbbell by slowly straightening your elbow to the starting position.

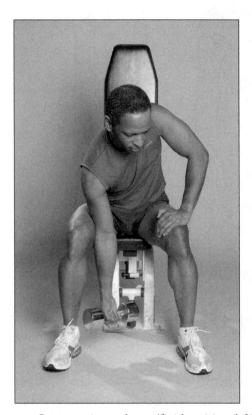 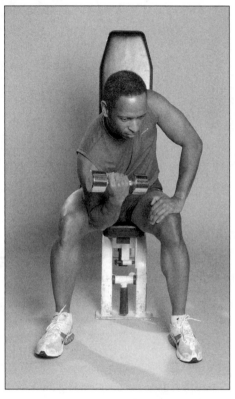

Concentration curl start/finish position (left). Concentration curl middle position (right).

Cable Curls

Cable curls are roughly equivalent to alternate dumbbell curls. They're good to do because they allow you to put constant tension on your muscle throughout the entire range of motion. Cable curls are also good because they give you a psychological change of pace.

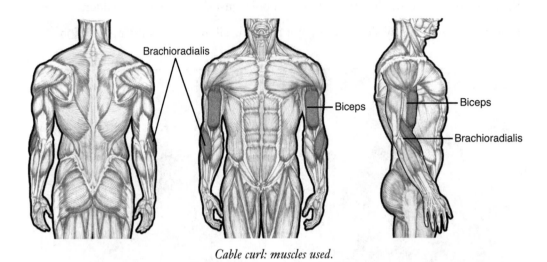

Cable curl: muscles used.

When performing a cable curl, **don't:**

- Lean backward to assist you in getting the weight up. If you need to do this before your last rep, reduce the weight instead.

- Allow the weight to bring your body forward as you lower it. If this happens, lighten the load.

SPOT ME

Although you will see people doing this exercise with both arms, we don't recommend it. Why? Doing bilateral bicep cable curls encourages you to arch your back. Unilateral bicep cable curls enable you to maintain proper posture during the exercise.

Do:

- Keep your abdomen tight and your knees slightly bent, to protect your back.

Here's how you properly perform a cable curl:

1. Grab hold of the handle from the bottom attachment of the cable crossover machine. (We'll show you more exercises you can do with cables later, in Chapter 14.) Different, interchangeable attachments are often used on cables. For this exercise, use a square-shaped handle.

2. Be sure your palm is facing inward, with your arm crossing your body slightly.

3. Stand with your feet shoulder width apart.

4. Slowly bend your elbow, stopping just short of your shoulder.

5. Slowly straighten your elbow, stopping just short of a fully straight position. The rhythm is the same here as for every other exercise: up for a 3-count and down for a 3-count.

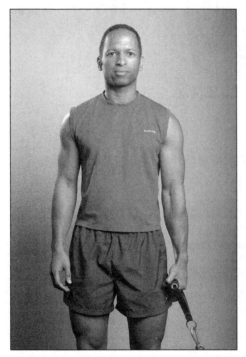 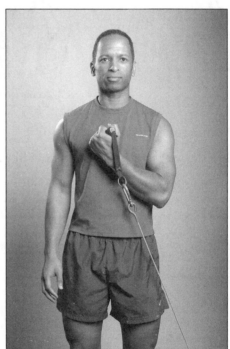

Cable curl start/finish position (left). Cable curl middle position (right).

Machine Curls

This exercise really isolates your biceps and makes it harder for you to cheat. The setup differs among machines, but the key is to fit yourself properly to avoid cheating.

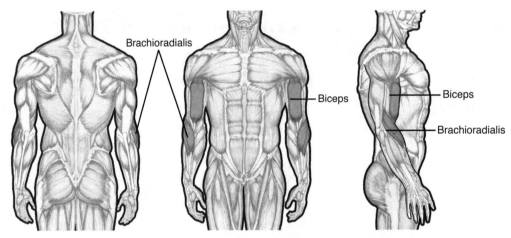

Machine curl: muscles used.

When performing a machine curl, **don't:**

- Allow the weight to bring you up out of the seat as you lower the weight.
- Hold your breath.

Do:

- Maintain good form, 3 counts up and 3 counts down.

Here's how you properly perform a machine curl:

1. Sit on the seat and place your arms on the pad. (Be sure that a trainer has shown you how to adjust the machine for a proper fit. A poor fit makes the exercise less effective and places more stress on your elbow and shoulder joints.)

2. Grab hold of the handles.

3. Keep your feet flat on the floor.

4. Slowly bend your elbows as far as you can; then slowly straighten your elbows, stopping just short of a fully straight position.

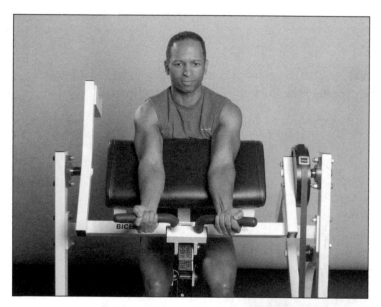

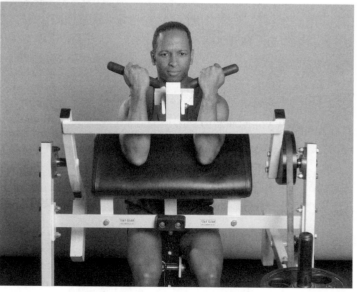

Machine curl start/finish position (top). Machine curl middle position (bottom).

Triceps

Typically, when we train biceps, we do exercises to work the triceps as well. Located in the back of your upper arm, the triceps and biceps are neighbors that share a backyard fence. The triceps are actually made of three muscles, hence the name. This triangular-shaped set of muscles is involved whenever you use your shoulders or chest in pressing, pushing movements.

Why strong triceps? For the following reasons:

* Your prowess at pushing a shopping cart (and other everyday activities) will improve.

* They look great and complement those new biceps of yours.

Triceps Kickbacks

The triceps kickback is a great way to isolate your triceps, but it requires strict form to be effective. You'll know you're doing it correctly when you feel the burn in the rear of your arm.

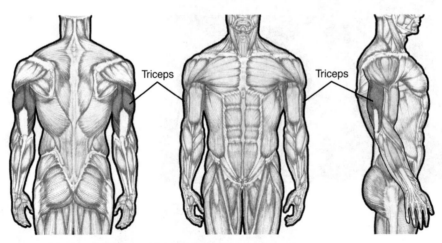

Triceps kickback: muscles used.

When performing a triceps kickback, **don't:**

* Allow your back to sag.

* Shift your body back and forth in an effort to get the weight up.

* Let your upper arm drop—keep it parallel to the ground throughout the range of motion.

Do:

* Keep your back straight and your abdomen tight.

* Keep your eyes fixed on the bench. Looking up or sideways can put stress on your neck.

Here's how you properly perform a triceps kickback:

1. Place one knee and one hand on the bench for support.

2. Slightly bend your standing leg.

3. Bend your working arm 90° at your shoulder and 90° at your elbow.

4. Keep your arm close to your side. To gain the full benefit from this exercise, it's important to keep your upper arm parallel to the ground. Pay strict attention to your form.

5. Slowly straighten your elbow and return to the starting position.

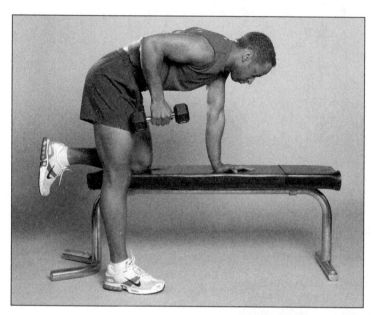

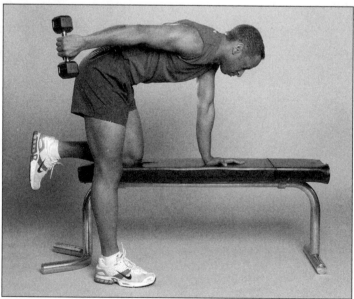

Triceps kickback start/finish position (top). Triceps kickback middle position (bottom).

French Curls

We're not sure why this particular exercise is identified with France, but feel free to do it regardless of your nationality. It's an excellent way to work your triceps.

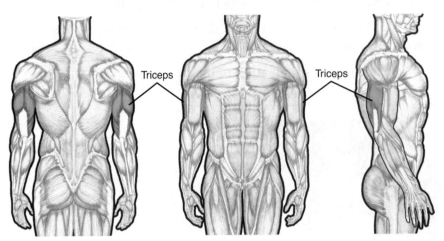

French curl: muscles used.

When performing a French curl, **don't:**

- Shift your body from side to side in an effort to raise the weight.
- Snap or lock your elbow upon straightening it.
- Allow the weight to fall rapidly to the starting position.

Do:

- Keep your abdomen tight, whether sitting or standing.
- Concentrate on your triceps and move gently through a full range of motion.

Here's how you properly perform a French curl:

1. While standing or sitting, raise the dumbbell overhead and bend your elbow to the point that you are feeling a stretch in your triceps.

2. Begin to straighten your elbow, and slowly return to your initial starting position.

> **WEIGHT A MINUTE**
>
> Be careful if you have been diagnosed with shoulder impingement syndrome (an abnormal squeezing of the structures within the shoulder joint). French curls can worsen the condition.

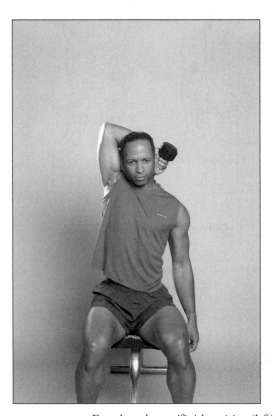 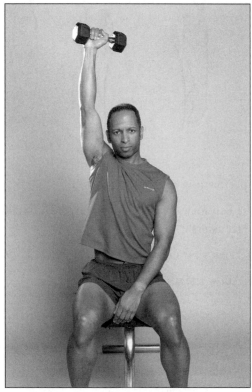

French curl start/finish position (left). French curl middle position (right).

Pushdowns

It's important to push hard at the bottom of the repetition to tighten (contract) your triceps. You can use either a rope or a bar attachment to perform this exercise; the rope is the harder of the two, and you typically use less weight than with the bar.

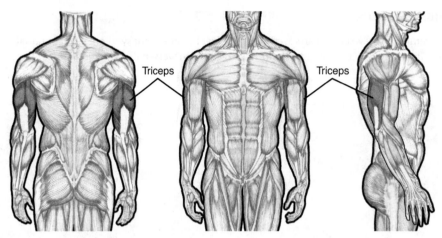

Pushdown: muscles used.

When performing a pushdown, **don't**:

- Lean forward as you push down the weight. This reduces the isolation from the triceps and transfers it to your whole body.
- Lock your elbows in the straightened position.
- Allow the weight to fall rapidly.

Do:

- Keep your abdomen tight and your back erect.
- Keep your head facing forward, not down or sideways.
- Keep your elbows close to your side.

Here's how you properly perform a pushdown:

1. Grab hold of the pushdown bar. Bend your elbows to 90° and hold them close to your side.

2. Slowly straighten your elbows and return to your initial starting position.

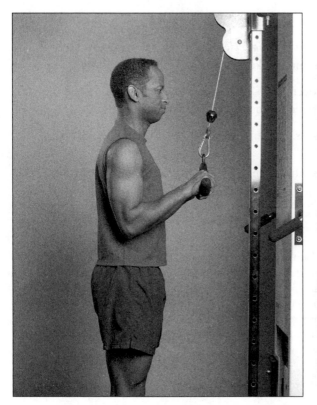 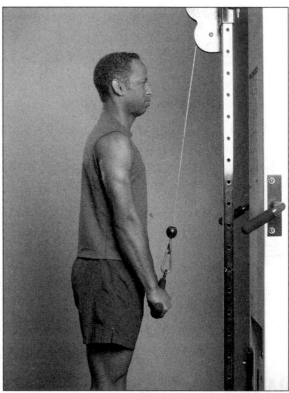

Pushdown start/finish position (left). Pushdown middle position (right).

Wrists

The muscles that work to bend and straighten your wrists actually originate at the elbow. In case you're curious, the muscles that bend (flex) the wrist originate in the inner part of the elbow. The muscles that straighten (extend) the wrist originate in the outer aspect of the elbow.

Why strong wrists? For the following reasons:

- Weak wrist muscles can lead to golfer's elbow *(medial epicondylitis)* or tennis elbow *(lateral epicondylitis)*. These injuries affect the pros and weekend warriors alike.

- Everyday activities like carrying heavy grocery bags or luggage can put strain on these muscles. In fact, people who use a screwdriver frequently suffer from tendinitis.

- If you care to embark on a career as a professional arm wrestler, you'll need strong wrists.

The best medicine is the preventive kind, which is why strengthening your wrists is important. A good way to avoid injuring your wrists is to do the following exercises.

WEIGHT A MINUTE

If you have carpal tunnel syndrome, do not perform these exercises because they're likely to aggravate it. This condition is often caused by repetitive activities done with improper body mechanics, such as typing with your wrists in an extended position (they should be neutral) or doing repetitive squeezing activities (as with what a cake decorator does when decorating a cake). The median nerve swells and is unable to pass comfortably through the small bones in the wrist (carpals). Symptoms of carpal tunnel syndrome are numbness, tingling, and a sharp, shooting pain into the hand.

Wrist Flexion

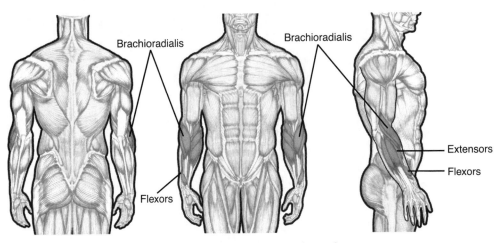

Wrist flexion/extension: muscles used.

Here's how you properly perform wrist flexion:

1. Lean forward.

2. Place your forearms on your thighs. Hold the dumbbell in a position past your knees, with your palm up.

3. Allow your wrist to bend as far back as you comfortably can.

4. Slowly bend your wrist up as far as you can; then return to the initial starting position.

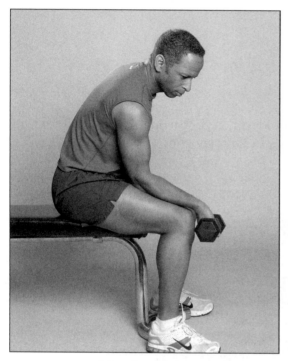 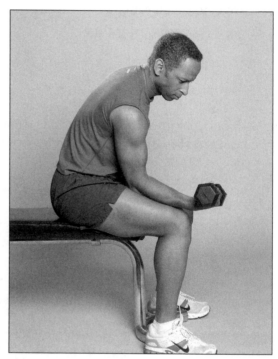

Wrist flexion start/finish position (left). Wrist flexion middle position (right).

Wrist Extension

Perform this exercise the same as you would the wrist flexion, but with your palms facing down.

When performing wrist flexion and extension, **don't**:

• Perform the movements rapidly in either direction.

Do:

• Keep your abdomen tight and your back erect.

Don't Do It

Building muscles in your arms can have both practical and aesthetic benefit, but don't let your desire for impressive arms get in the way of your good sense.

Once again, cheating makes it much easier to move more weight. That's great for your ego but not so much for your back. More to the point, it's not helping build strong arms. Avoid these common but crucial mistakes in your biceps exercises:

- Arching your back
- Holding your breath
- Throwing your pelvis forward
- Raising your elbows
- Moving the bar too fast

Bulging biceps look great, but just throwing a ton of weight on the bar and getting the bar up any way you can isn't the safest or most effective way to get those "big guns." Here's another "Don't Do It" for you.

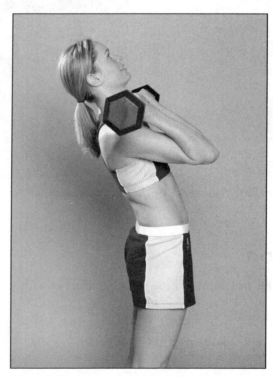

What's wrong with this picture? Try the arched back, raised elbows, and forward pelvis to start.

Keep your shoulders over your hips and your hips over your ankles. Don't let your elbows rise during the exercise—that involves your shoulders and does your biceps no good.

Gut Buster

In This Chapter

- Comparing abs versus flab
- Understanding the rectus abdominis
- Losing the midsection myths
- Joining the washboard world

Here's a bit of abdominal irony to ponder: as a nation, we seem to loathe fat people even though we're the most overweight nation in the Western world. A portly belly might have been a sign of prosperity in the Far East, but in our culture, a flat stomach is a prized possession, despite the fact that most people refuse to do what it takes to get there.

Socioeconomic implications aside, there are several solid reasons to build a washboard stomach:

- It looks good.
- It will make you feel better, especially if you have an ailing back.
- You'll be stronger in the weight room and on the playing field.

Before we give you the lowdown on building up your midsection, let's review our anatomy. The first and most common mistake is referring to the abdominals (the "abs") as "the stomach." The abs are the muscles in your midsection; your stomach is the organ that processes the food you consume. Ab exercises have traditionally included sit-ups and leg lifts; stomach exercises include dining in a French restaurant.

Your abdominals consist of four muscles:

- The *rectus abdominis*, the largest muscle in the abs, is a wide, flat sheet of muscle that runs from just under the lower part of your chest to just below your belly button. When you do abdominal crunches, the old rectus abdominis muscle is hard at work. (For more on crunches, read on.) It also keeps your spine from slip-sliding around when you're exercising other body parts.

- The *internal obliques* and *external obliques*, which run diagonally along your sides, not only assist the rectus in curling the spine, but also twist and bend your upper body. These muscles are central in any sport involving upper-body rotation—golf, baseball, kayaking, and many more—and they are integral in a strengthening program, especially if you have a bad back. Why? These muscles wrap around your waist and, when properly conditioned, provide much-needed support for your lower back. In essence, the obliques are the world's most comfortable form-fitting girdle.

- The *transversus abdominis*, which sounds like a phrase from a Latin Mass, is the deepest of all the muscles in your abs. Located directly below the rectus abdominis, it is called into action when you sneeze, cough, or exhale forcefully. You don't do specific exercises to target this muscle, but you can strengthen the transversus abdominis by forcefully exhaling during the positive phase of your ab exercises.

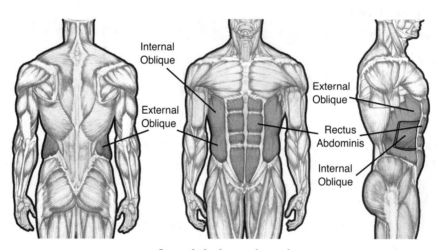

Lateral plank: muscles used.

Feel the Burn

As we've mentioned, having strong abs significantly helps you get rid of lower back pain. Try this: sit in a chair. Hold your abs tight. Now let them go. Did you note a difference in your posture? You see, your abs are what keep your pelvis in a neutral position. When your abs are weak, your pelvis has a tendency to tilt forward, increasing the inward curve of your lumbar spine. This, of course, throws the rest of your spine out of whack as well. All you have to do to see what we're talking about is check out the exaggerated curve of someone with a sizeable beer belly. Contrast that, say, with the posture of an athlete such as an Olympic gymnast, and you can begin to see the relationship in strong abs, good posture, and improved athletic performance.

Perhaps because there's so much discussion and even obsession with our bulging waistlines, a lot of misinformation surrounds the abs. We'd like to clear it up.

Here are a few of the most common midsection myths:

- **"If I work my abs, I'll get rid of my love handles."** This is the one we hear most often. You can do 5,000 sit-ups a day, but because the muscle lies beneath the fat, these muscles will function efficiently but not be seen. In other words, strong abs and love handles have nothing to do with each other. Want to lose the excess baggage? Eat less and do more cardiovascular exercise.

- **"I need to do 500 crunches a day to get my abs in really great shape."** If you can do 500 crunches a day, either you're a Navy SEAL in training or you're doing something quite wrong. (More often than not, it's the latter.) Done correctly, 10 to 25 repetitions for three sets is more than enough to get the job done. Why waste your time by doing so many, especially if you do them incorrectly?

- **"I do my abs every day for maximum benefit."** This is another line we hear a lot in the gym. The abs can be worked more than your chest or biceps, for example, but you should treat your abs as you treat any other muscles. They need rest just like any other stressed body part. Working them more often does not improve results.

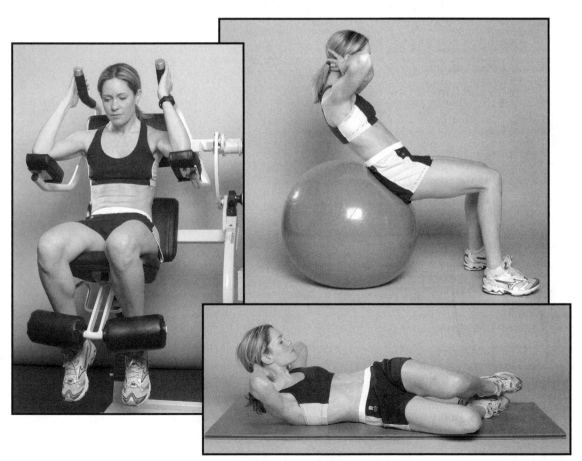

Some of the exercises in this chapter.

Planks

Though it may not look particularly impressive, the plank is one of the most effective exercises for building strength and endurance in the abdominals, lower back, and other supporting core muscles.

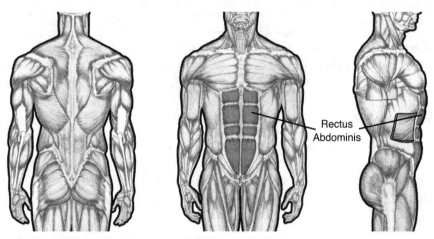

Rectus
Abdominis

Plank: muscles used.

When doing a plank, **don't:**

- Let your body drop.
- Hold your breath.

Do:

- Keep your abs contracted.
- Gradually increase the amount of time you hold the position.

Here's the drill:

1. Lie face down.

2. Raise onto your toes and forearms.

3. Keep your body in a straight line from head to heels.

4. Hold the position.

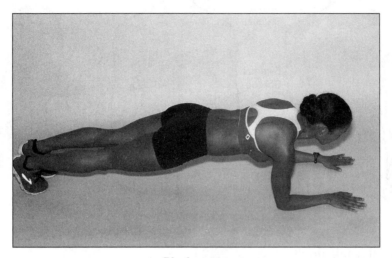

Plank position.

Lateral Planks

As the name suggests, the lateral plank is much like its supine counterpart, but this time you're on your side. Like the standard plank, it's a great exercise for developing core strength and stability. And while it's not easy, it is simple.

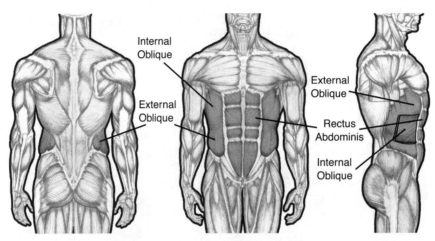

Lateral plank: muscles used.

When doing a lateral plank, **don't:**

- Let your body sink.
- Clench your jaw or tense muscles not in use.

Do:

- Breathe normally.
- Gradually increase the time you hold the position.

1. Lie on your side, with your elbow and forearm on the ground.

2. Stack your feet one on top of the other.

3. Lift your body in a straight line.

4. Raise the top arm toward the ceiling.

5. Turn your head to the ceiling.

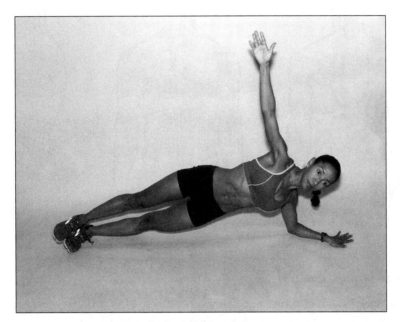

Lateral plank position.

Crunches

If you're stuck on a desert island with just one ab exercise, crunches are the one. Done properly, you're bound to feel a nice burn in no time flat.

Initially, the exercise feels rather easy; however, after several reps, you should begin to feel a burn in the upper third of your abs.

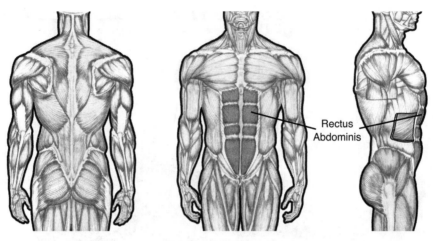

Rectus
Abdominis

Crunches: muscles used.

When performing a crunch, **don't:**

- Bend your neck as you curl into the crunch position. This is the biggest reason that people who do a lot of ab work complain. Imagine having a softball between your chin and your chest.

- Draw your elbows in. You're trying to lift your torso, not flap your elbows.

- Bring your torso up past 30°.

WEIGHT A MINUTE

Be sure not to "throw" your head forward when doing crunches. To avoid causing neck pain, your hands should support your head and you should maintain space between your chin and your chest.

Do:

- Keep your head and neck in a neutral position; the less stress on your neck, the better.

- Be sure you curl as you lift.

- Focus your attention on the top section of your abdominals. Let them—and not any other part of your upper body—do the work.

- Keep your lower back pressed against the floor at all times.

Here's how you properly perform a crunch:

1. Lie on a mat with your knees bent and your feet on the floor. Depending on your level of fitness, you can place your arms in any of the three following positions:

   Beginner: Keep your arms straight at your sides and point your fingers toward your knees.

   Intermediate: Cross your arms over your chest.

   Advanced: Bend your elbows and overlap your fingers behind your neck.

2. Tighten your stomach muscles and slowly curl your torso up until your shoulder blades are off the floor.

3. Slowly return to your starting position without completely relaxing on the floor.

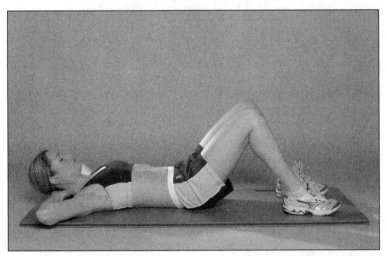

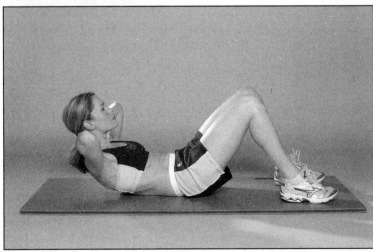

Crunch start/finish position (top). Crunch middle position (bottom).

Reverse Crunches

Here's a tricky one that takes some time to get used to. It's not nearly as impressive-looking as some of the crazy leg lifts and other things you'll see people doing in an effort to strengthen their lower abs, but it's far more safe and effective.

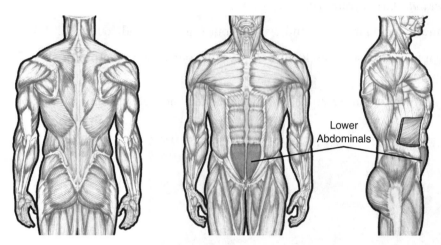

Lower
Abdominals

Reverse crunches: muscles used.

When performing a reverse crunch, **don't**:

- Roll your hips so your back comes off the mat.
- Tighten your shoulders or involve any upper-body movement.
- Hold your breath. (People always seem to on this exercise.)

Do:

- Keep the movement small—no need to roll back, too.
- Keep the movement smooth.
- Isolate the muscle by concentrating on the lower section of your abs.

SPOT ME

Because your abdominal muscles assist when you forcefully exhale, breathing out during the positive phase of your ab exercises helps you get an even better contraction.

Here's how you properly perform a reverse crunch:

1. Lie on a mat with your legs up and your knees slightly bent. In the starting position, you'll look like a big letter L.

2. Rest your arms on the floor at your sides.

3. Keep your head on the mat and tighten your abdominals.

4. Lift your butt off the floor so that your legs go up and slightly backward toward your head.

5. Hold this position for a second and slowly return to the starting position.

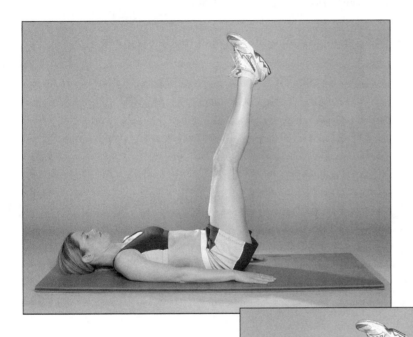

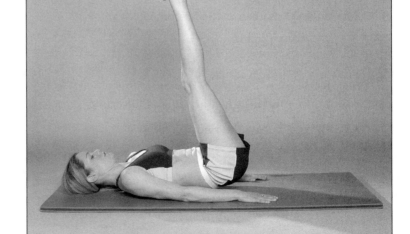

Reverse crunch start/finish position (top). Reverse crunch middle position (bottom).

Ball Crunches

The ball crunch is a variation on the standard crunch and is performed on an oversized orb called a *Swiss ball* or a *stability ball*. The ball is obviously less stable than a mat and forces you to use small stabilizing muscles in your midsection to help maintain balance.

DEFINITION

Swiss balls, or **stability balls,** are large, inflatable rubber balls used for abdominal and other exercises. They come in different sizes, with a 55-inch diameter recommended for those under 5 feet, 5 inches; 65 inches for those up to 6 feet tall; and 75 inches for people taller than 6 feet.

The form is largely the same as with the crunch, although the range of motion is great.

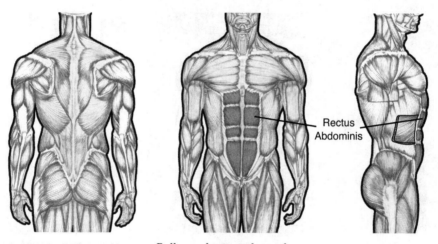

Rectus Abdominis

Ball crunches: muscles used.

When doing the ball crunch, **don't:**

- Bounce off the ball at the bottom.
- Thrust your head forward.

Do:

- Contract your abs when lifting and lowering.
- Keep your feet on the floor.

Here's the drill:

1. Sit on the high section of the ball with your feet flat on the floor, hip width apart. Lie back on the ball. Place your hands in the same position as in the crunch.

2. Contract your abdominal muscles and raise your torso off the ball until your shoulder blades and midback are clear.

3. Slowly lower yourself back onto the ball, keeping your abs tight at all times.

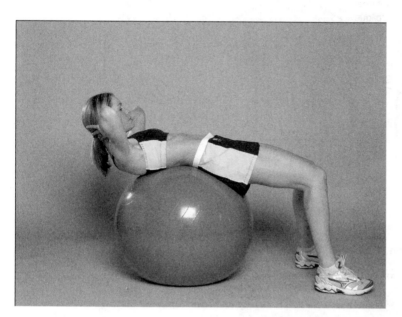

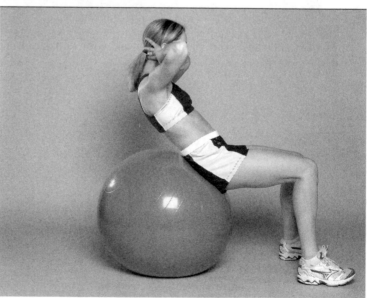

Ball crunch start/finish position (top). Ball crunch middle position (bottom).

Oblique Crunches

Here's another one that's commonly abused in the gym. Focus on moving your shoulder toward your opposite knee. Avoid the temptation to move your elbow in or your knee back.

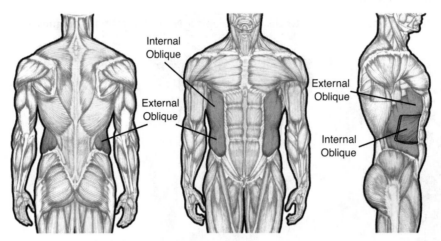

Oblique crunches: muscles used.

When performing an oblique crunch, **don't:**

- Bend your head with your hand.
- Merely move your elbow to your knee.

Do:

- Curl and twist your shoulder toward your opposite knee.
- Keep the movement slow and controlled.

Here's how you properly perform an oblique crunch:

1. Lie on a mat with your left leg bent and your foot flat on the floor.

2. Place your right ankle so that it rests on top of your left knee.

3. Position your left hand behind your neck, and keep your right arm outstretched.

4. Slowly curl up and twist toward your right knee.

5. Hold that position for a second and then slowly return to the starting position.

6. Switch legs and arms, and repeat on the other side.

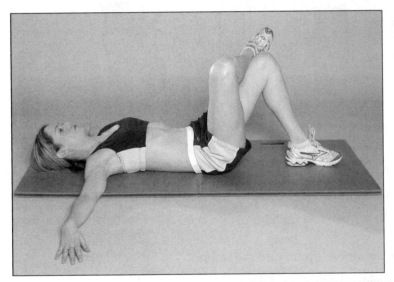

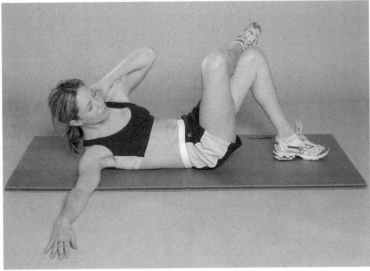

Oblique crunch start/finish position (top). Oblique crunch middle position (bottom).

Side Obliques

Here's an alternative to the previous exercise. Use it to break up the monotony whenever you please. If you choose this exercise, be sure to keep your knees to the side to keep the focus on your obliques.

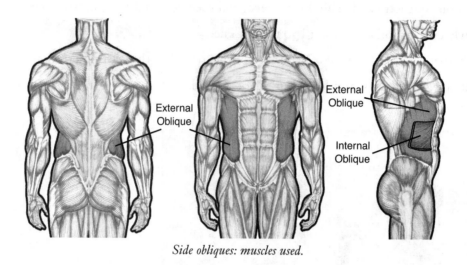

Side obliques: muscles used.

When performing a side oblique, **don't:**

- Bend your neck to the side as you lift your torso off the mat.

Do:

- Keep your shoulder and head going straight toward the ceiling.
- Be sure your knees stay to the side.

Here's how you properly perform a side oblique:

1. Lie on a mat on your right side with your knees bent.

2. Place both hands behind your neck, and keep your head looking straight at the ceiling.

3. Use your oblique muscles to lift your upper body slightly off the mat.

4. Hold yourself off the mat for a second and then return to your starting position.

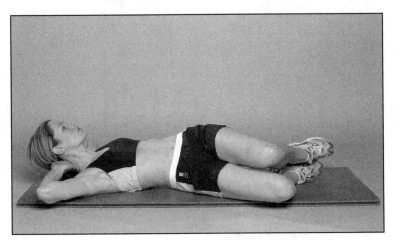

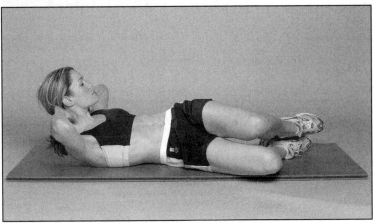

Side oblique start/finish position (top). Side oblique middle position (bottom).

Machine Crunches

To isolate your abdomen, slowly move the arm pad toward your knees using the muscles in your upper abs. Pause for a second at the bottom of the repetition and return to the starting position without completely releasing the tension in your abs.

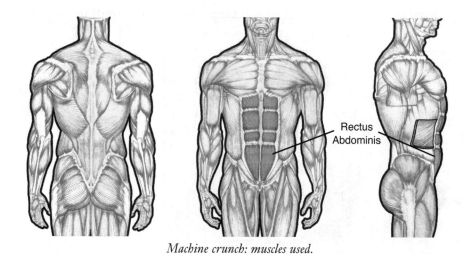

Rectus
Abdominis

Machine crunch: muscles used.

When performing a machine crunch, **don't:**

- Use too much weight so your hips are lifted off the seat.
- Let the weights you're lifting slam down on the stack.
- Arch your back as you return to the starting position.
- Focus on pushing the arm pad down; rather, concentrate on curling your abdomen.

Do:

- Keep constant tension on your abdominals as you perform the exercise.

Here's how you properly perform a machine crunch:

1. Sit on the seat and fasten the belt, if one is provided.

2. Place your arms on top of the arm pad.

3. Slowly tighten your abdominal muscles, curling your torso forward. As you do this, you'll be bringing the arm pad toward your thighs.

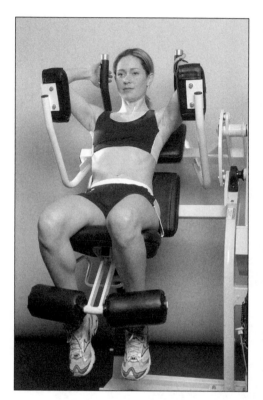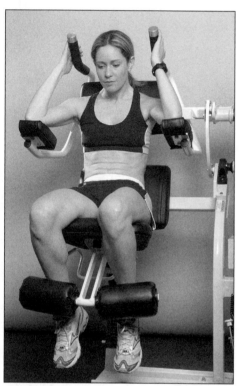

Machine crunch start/finish position (left). Machine crunch middle position (right).

Get with the Program

In This Chapter

- Putting it all together
- Knowing when sore is good
- Understanding when too much is bad
- Being bored no more

You've read this far, and you no doubt know more than you ever wanted to know about form, safety, sets, and reps, as well as a slew of fancy words that ensure you know the difference between your lats and your pecs. In addition, you're now familiar with the mechanics of a host of exercises to keep you busy until the next millennium. What you might not know, however, is how to put it all together. Having all the ingredients for a soufflé is one thing; knowing how to assemble them is another. In this chapter, we show you how to use the information we've discussed thus far to build a workout routine fit for a hungry king.

As we've mentioned, if you talk to a dozen fitness experts, you're liable to get half a dozen or more opinions on how much to lift, how often, and more. Although virtually everyone will tell you to progress from larger muscles to smaller muscles, the wide variety of opinions can be quite confusing. We can't say that everyone who dares to disagree with us has a head full of iron, but we can tell you that if you follow what we suggest in this chapter and the chapters that follow, you'll get stronger and also look and feel better. If you're skeptical, try one of the following routines and see for yourself.

Finally, we realize that not all gyms are created equal. As a result, you may not have all the equipment we demonstrated at your disposal. To account for this athletic inequity, we've included a few different basic workout plans to get you started.

What to Do

When you look over the programs in this chapter, your first reaction may be that they don't include a lot of exercises. There's a reason for this. Because we're asking you to work hard and exhibit perfect form on each, as a trade-off, we don't ask you to do a lot of exercises. After all, it's only human that your concentration and willpower will falter if you have to do an endless series of exercises each time. As we promised throughout the book, working out needn't take you all day.

These basic routines shouldn't take more than 45 minutes each. That includes about 1 minute for each of the exercises and 2 minutes off between each set. That's not a significant investment in time, but if you do these routines faithfully—with effort and concentration—you'll get stronger. As you can see from the following chart, we've imitated a Chinese menu (one from Column A, one from Column B) and tried to give you the option of deciding between free weights and machine exercises whenever possible. Depending on your preference and the availability of any one machine or free weight apparatus, there's no need to stick with one exclusively.

Whenever you see an exercise highlighted in **bold,** that means we want you to do a light warm-up set with about half your normal weight before moving on to your regular set of these exercises. Remember to aim for sets of 10 to 12 reps with a 3-second positive and 3-second negative, with a 1-second pause between. In other words, lifting the weight takes 3 seconds, the downward phase takes 3 seconds, and so on until the set is done. Take 2 minutes between exercises. You can take less time, if you care to, but try hard not to take more. If you do, that 45-minute figure will creep over the 1-hour mark.

Here's a chart to help you pick one of the following exercises from the machine column and/or free weight column. Feel free to mix it up—use some free weight exercises and some machines, if you like. Work your way from the top of the list to the bottom.

Mix-and-Match Machines and Free Weights

Muscle	Machine Exercise	Free Weight Exercise
Glutes, quads, hamstrings	**Leg press**	**Lunges**
Quads	Leg extension	
Hamstrings	Leg curl	
Gastroc (calves)	Standing toe raise	
Lats	**Lat pull-down**	**Pull-ups** (assisted, if necessary)
Traps	Shrug	
Pecs	**Chest press**	**Bench press**
Flye	Pec deck	
Delts	Shoulder press Lateral raise	Dumbbell military press Lateral raise
Biceps	Biceps machine	Seated dumbbell curl
Triceps	Triceps push-down	French curl
Abs	Abdominal machine	Crunches
Obliques	Cable rotations	Oblique crunches
Lower back	Back raise	

Keeping Track

Your main goal during the first few weeks is to learn to do the exercises properly. At the same time, it's important to keep track of what you're doing. That's where a workout log comes in. We don't want to make this seem like preparing your income taxes. However, keeping accurate records of your workouts not only helps you track your progress, but is also a great way to figure out what to do when you hit a plateau. Getting stronger requires that you overload your muscles; as a result, it's key that you know what you've done in previous workouts. If you're anything like us, you'll actually find it fun to see how much progress you've made in a relatively short amount of time.

Your workout log should list everything you've done that day in the gym—your choice of exercises, how much weight, how many reps—as well as the height of the seat on the machines you're using. It's also a good idea to note how you were feeling on that day, your body weight, and any other relevant facts. In time, you'll see that this physical record is a diary that accurately reflects the relationships among your mental, physical, and emotional lives. In fact, the more carefully you note the impact of outside factors on your lifting, the more you're likely to see a powerful relationship forming in how all facets of your life affect your weight training.

I'm Late! I'm Late!

Of course, in this busy world where time is often money, even 45 minutes can seem like too much time to spare. If that's the case for you, don't worry. It's far better to work out just a little than not at all. Let's say you want to squeeze in a workout at lunch and still have time to shower and grab a bite. Or perhaps you want to run a couple miles and you have just 20 minutes or so to lift afterward. No matter—we give you a condensed workout to keep you on track. These shorter workouts are not as thorough as the longer versions, and they're better suited to maintaining strength than getting you stronger, but they take care of the basics. Just as important, they ensure that you won't lose fitness.

The shorter workout is essentially the same as the longer one. The biggest difference is that each of these exercises is a *multijoint* or *compound movement*, meaning that you'll be working at least two joints, and thus more muscles, during any one lift. *Single-joint* or *isolation movements* like the flye (chest) or lateral raise (shoulder) are great, but you don't cover as much ground with each exercise.

DEFINITION

Multijoint or **compound movements** are exercises that involve two or more joints. **Single-joint** or **isolation** movements use only one. Compound movements like the bench press or squat use more musculature and generally result in the weight moving in a fairly straight line, whereas isolation moves like the flye or leg extension focus on a specific muscle and usually have a rotary movement.

Perform a light warm-up set of the bold exercises. Reduce your recovery time between sets from 2 minutes to 1. Done correctly, you're in and out in less than 15 minutes. Remember that even if you're in a hurry, don't perform your reps quickly just for the sake of time. Focus on proper form, and get as much out of each and every rep as you can. The key here is intensity.

The following table can be your quickie guide to a great 15-minute workout.

15-Minute Workout

Muscle	Exercise
Glutes, hamstrings, quads	Leg press
Lats	Lat pull-down or pull-ups
Pecs	Bench press or dips
Traps	Upright rows
Delts	Shoulder press
Abs	Crunches

Progress Report

Let's say that you've done every rep of every set with perfect form. Let's also assume that you warm up and stretch religiously, and your nutrition is as pure as a field of soybeans. No doubt you will discover that, regardless of how slowly you started your program, you've had your share of aches and pains. If you're wondering whether this is normal, the answer is "Yes." The bottom line is that, although we do everything we can to help you avoid injuries, muscle soreness is a natural consequence of a new weightlifting program.

Whenever you introduce a new activity to your body, you experience what we call growing pains. This is a natural consequence as your muscles, tendons, and ligaments adapt to the new stresses and strains of muscular overload. In fact, even someone who is ridiculously fit will be sore after doing a new routine with any intensity. We want you to be able to differentiate between *good* hurt and *bad* hurt. Good hurt you can work through; bad hurt is a sure signal to stop immediately.

You're likely to experience two types of soreness during weight training: acute soreness—the discomfort you feel during and right after a set—and a more gradual, duller ache that comes on in the days after you lift.

The Burn

In gym parlance, acute soreness is referred to as "the burn." Typically, it occurs during and immediately following exercise. When you're completing the last few reps of a set, your muscles are working hard. As the muscle is taxed, it actually presses against your arteries and cuts off blood flow. (This is the rough equivalent of wearing an inflated cuff when you're having your blood pressure taken.) As a result, lactic acid, a byproduct of anaerobic activity, accumulates. This combination of lactic acid and blood flow occlusion is thought to cause momentary muscle failure. Got that? The miracle of the human body is that, within a few seconds of the end of the set, the burn dissipates as the muscle is engorged with even more blood than usual to compensate for what was lost during the set. This process causes the temporary (but ego-boosting) "pump" phenomenon.

The DOMS

Delayed onset muscle soreness (DOMS) refers to the pain and soreness that occurs 24 to 48 hours after exercise. DOMS results from the microscopic muscle damage that takes place when you lift. The eccentric or negative phase of the exercise contributes more than its fair share to this soreness. Usually, you'll feel the beginning of DOMS the day after you lift; however, it often reaches its peak at about 48 hours after the fact. Putting ice on the affected area can help reduce some of the edema (or retention of water) at the site and alleviate the pain. The soreness should start to ease after that and last no more than three to four days. If the pain lasts significantly longer or becomes worse, we recommend that you see a physician.

SPOT ME

We've given you a number of reasons to stretch, but alleviating delayed onset muscle soreness is not one of them. Despite gym lore, stretching doesn't speed your recovery from DOMS. Studies have shown that although increased flexibility may help prevent or decrease the incidence of soreness in the first place, when you're sore, stretching isn't going to help.

That Hurts!

A burn during a set and soreness afterward is as common as a pigeon in a park. Although the term *good pain* may be a classic oxymoron, normal pains are definitely associated with the weightlifting game. Of course, some types of pain are not normal and shouldn't be taken lightly. In fact, unless you've been doing it a long while, the old bromide of "No pain, no gain" is generally considered passé and counterproductive.

Here's the bottom line: any sharp and shooting pain is bad, no matter where it occurs. Such an acute sensation indicates nerve pain and should send an immediate warning. Pain that occurs in any of your joints (shoulder, elbow, wrist, hip, knee, or ankle) is also a red flag. As we've stressed all along, be mindful of your form and of the amount of weight you're lifting.

FLEX FACTS

Lactic acid is usually to blame when you feel a burning sensation during your lift or while sprinting to catch a bus, but it's just an innocent bystander when it comes to DOMS. Even after a brutal workout, your lactic acid levels return to normal within a couple hours of a workout.

If your form is not sound, you put additional stress on your joints simply because you are putting your body in a position it doesn't want to be in. This means that even if you were performing the exercise with just your body weight, you would experience some pain and discomfort. Add a barbell to the equation, and you're bound to aggravate the situation. It sounds so simple, but time and time again, we see people lifting heavy weights with chronically injured joints. Determination clearly has a place in the gym, but when it's misapplied, it's a sure way to court serious injury.

WEIGHT A MINUTE

A burning sensation is normal during a challenging set of weightlifting, and soreness over the next couple days is not unusual. However, any sharp or shooting pain while lifting is a red flag to stop immediately. If this occurs, never try to fight through such pain. Review your form to be sure you're not doing anything wrong. If your form isn't at fault, try another exercise that works the same body part.

Let's take a look at a couple broad categories and discuss how to best treat them.

Pulls and Strains

Minor muscle pulls or muscle *strains* are a common injury associated with weightlifting. With careful attention to proper technique and caution against using too much weight, you usually can avoid strains.

Sprains are another common injury, although they are usually avoidable. Moderate strains and sprains are usually treated in the same way—with rest, ice, compression, and elevation, or RICE. Here are the specifics:

- **Rest.** Eliminates the demands on the affected area. If you can't rest it entirely, at least modify it as much as possible. (That would be MICE.)

- **Ice.** Decreases swelling, pain, and circulation.

- **Compression.** Limits swelling with the pressure of a bandage.

- **Elevation.** Reduces or limits swelling by reducing blood flow to the injured area.

DEFINITION

A muscle **strain** or pull is a trauma to the muscle or tendon caused by excessive contraction or stretching. **Sprains** are damage to ligaments (ligaments are the connective tissue between bones) accompanied by swelling and sometimes discoloration.

Overtraining

Overtraining can be another source of aches and pains. It's also a factor that may inhibit muscular strength gains. Symptoms of overtraining include the following:

- Chronic fatigue
- Appetite disorders
- Sleeplessness
- Depression
- Anger
- Substantial weight gain or loss
- Protracted muscle soreness
- Elevated resting heart rate
- Lack of progress in muscular strength

If you are experiencing any of these symptoms with your weightlifting program, perhaps you began too ambitiously. In our experience, the two most common symptoms of overtraining are an uncomfortable night's sleep and moodiness. Listen to your body, rest, and begin again at a more modest pace.

DEFINITION

Overtraining occurs when you train without allowing sufficient recovery between workouts or when you do too much too fast. Sometimes it rears its ugly head with physical symptoms, and sometimes it's mental. Usually a couple extra days off will help remedy the situation.

If you've been lifting consistently, don't worry that a few extra days off will hurt your strength. Many of Jonathan's most dedicated clients travel quite a bit—either for work or for pleasure. Often he tells them to relax and not work out on the road. Much to their surprise, they actually benefit from the short break, and they're stronger than ever when they return.

When she was competing as a powerlifter, our sage expert Deidre was a poster child for overtraining. Not only did she not stretch, but she also worked out every single day, whether she was lifting weights or doing cardiovascular exercise. She looked great, but she was an achy mess most of the time, especially in the morning, when she struggled to get out of bed with a chronically sore lower back. During her last year of competition in 1997, she was hurt more often than not and was frequently depressed and disagreeable. If her coach said the sky was up, she'd argue otherwise. Such is the nature of a compulsive world champion, but it's not necessary (or even helpful) for general health.

This Isn't Working

When it comes to weight training, it takes at least six weeks of consistent training to begin to notice physical changes in your body. That's six weeks of *consistent* training. Often people think they're training intensely when, in fact, they're pushing themselves while they lift but taking a ton of time between sets. In other words, be sure you're following our guidelines before you assume that you're making little or no progress. However, if after six weeks of diligent gym work you don't notice a change—even if it's slight—you may consider tinkering with your routine. A few ways you may alter your routine are as follows:

- **Vary the number of reps.** Generally, we like a range of 10 to 12, but that's not written in stone. Try decreasing the weight by 5 to 10 percent, and bump up your rep range to 12 to 15.

- **Decrease the amount of rest between sets.** If you are resting for 2 minutes, decrease it to 1 minute. You'll probably have to decrease the weight by a few pounds, but you'll find it really challenging.

- **Change the exercises.** Most free weight exercises we showed you have machine equivalents, and vice versa. Try mixing it up for a while. Remember, the more you keep your muscles guessing, the better off you are.

To make gains in strength and in your appearance, you must continue to put stress on your muscles. If you are constantly doing sets of 10 reps with 10-pound biceps curls when you could clearly do an eleventh repetition, you're not going to see much of a change. Getting strong means using as many muscle fibers as possible during your exercise. The last few reps should be difficult. Once it becomes easy, you must increase the stress on the muscle by upping the weight you lift—that is, if you want to get stronger.

I'm Bored

No matter what the activity, weight training can get pretty boring if you're doing the same thing every time you hit the gym. Even if you increase the weight/reps or decrease your rest, if the basis of your routine is the same, you can become mentally tired. This is when you need to play around with some special techniques that can add a much-needed jolt to your program.

If you find that, despite hard efforts, you don't appear to be getting stronger over the course of three to four weeks, it may be time for a rest or a change in your program. If you're exhibiting any of the signs of overtraining we outlined earlier, try taking a few extra days off. If you feel good but have just hit a plateau, you can try varying the program.

Changing a program every few months helps avoid mental boredom, but it also helps keep your muscles challenged. By varying the exercises from time to time, you ensure that you present new challenges for your muscles. Even making a subtle change in angle from a free weight exercise to its machine equivalent or switching from a barbell to dumbbells can give a muscle a little surprise and help push you through plateaus.

You can tinker with your exercise plan in countless ways. In the next few chapters, we show you some advanced techniques you can use to spice up your program.

The Least You Need to Know

- Now that you've learned the basics, it's time to assemble a solid routine.
- You can make tremendous gains in only 45 minutes a day.
- No matter how good your form, stiff and sore muscles are par for the course.
- Being enthusiastic is great; doing too much, too often can be bad.
- Changing your routine is great for your muscles and ensures that you won't be bored.

Balls, Bells, and Cables

In This Chapter

- Strength training using the kettlebell
- Building fitness and preventing injuries with the medicine ball
- Using cables to build more functional fitness

Back when Greece wasn't ancient, Hippocrates—that famous physician best remembered for his Oath—had his patients working out with medicine balls made of animal skins filled with sand. Unlike their modern counterpart, which are made of leather or vinyl, this ancient fitness tool has become a standard piece of equipment in gyms across the country.

Flash-forward a few thousand years to the kettlebell, another prime example of this back-to-the-future trend in fitness. Favored by Russian weightlifters more than a century ago, these no-frills weights, which look like a cannonball with a thick handle but behave like the world's most unwieldy iron tea kettle, are even more versatile than the medicine ball. Because the weight of the kettlebell sits just below a thick handle, "controlling" the weight requires you to use more muscle groups and, as they say in Vladivostok, ups the fitness bang for your ruble.

That leads us to the third core-centric, frequently ignored category of exercise: cable training. Cable training might not predate Hercules, but unlike regular strength-training equipment, which is high on isolating a particular muscle, cables require more coordination and, consequently, force you to use more muscle groups per exercise. We've already shown you a few cable exercises in earlier chapters; here we show you some other ways to take advantage of their versatility. "Multiplanar movements are desirable because the body is designed to move as a unit," says Damon Roxas, national director of personal training for Crunch Fitness in New York City. Said more simply, you're working your muscles as they actually function when you're outside running, jumping, or chasing a bus with groceries.

While we still favor getting started with dumbbells, barbells, and machines, incorporating kettle-bells, medicine balls, and cables into your training regimen can take your training to new heights.

Why Kettlebells?

The asymmetrical construction of the kettlebell makes it difficult to control. Not only does it improve your hand strength, but your core has to work harder than if you were using a dumbbell. Couple that with exercises that target the whole body, and you have a formula for significant strength gains in minimal time. You can do scores of exercises with kettlebells, but for now, we introduce a couple of the most basic and important.

FLEX FACTS

Kettlebell training burns a surprisingly high number of calories. A study by the American Council on Exercise found that a 20-minute kettlebell workout burns about 21 calories a minute, the equivalent of running at a 6-minute-mile pace.

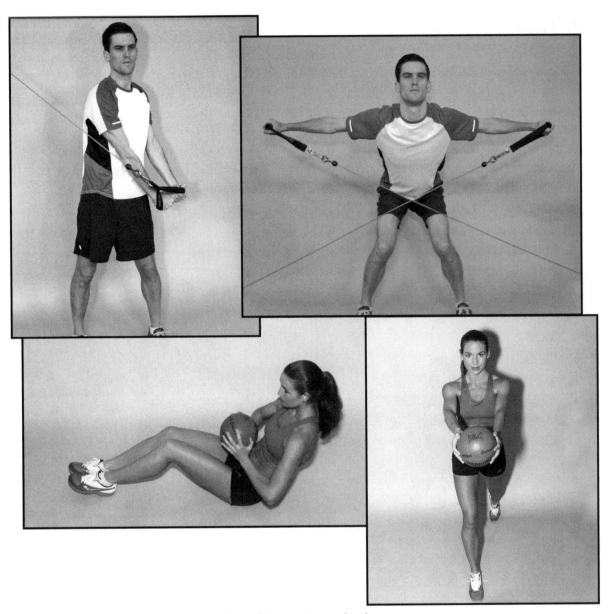

Some of the exercises in this chapter.

Swings

Keep in mind that although this may look like a shoulder exercise, it really works your hips, legs, and core. Your arm is just along for the ride, as the hip initiates the movement. Swings also work great with both arms together on one kettlebell.

1. Stand with your feet shoulder width apart.

2. Squat to pick up the kettlebell with one arm.

3. Exhale, initiating an upward movement to swing the kettlebell upward until your arm is parallel to the ground, while you return to a standing position.

4. Keeping your arm straight, let the kettlebell fall between your legs as you return to your squatting position.

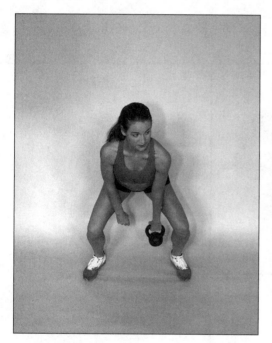 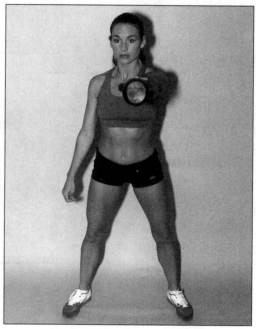

Kettlebell swings start/finish position (left). Kettlebell swings middle position (right).

Squat and Press

Gene Schaffer, an athletic trainer at ARC Athletics in New York, calls this his "desert island kettlebell exercise" because you work practically every major muscle in your body when you do it.

1. Begin with a wide stance, holding the round section of the kettlebell with the handle down. (This is sometimes referred to as the "goblet position.") Keep your elbows in and the kettlebell against your chest.

2. Squat, keeping the kettlebell against your chest.

3. As you come up from the squat, begin to press the kettlebell overhead.

4. Continue to press the kettlebell upward after you complete the squat.

5. Return to the squatting position as you bring the kettlebell back down to your chest.

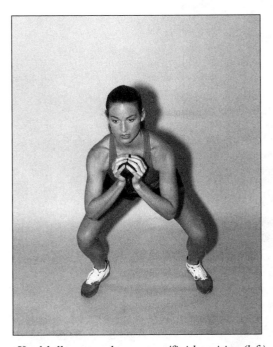 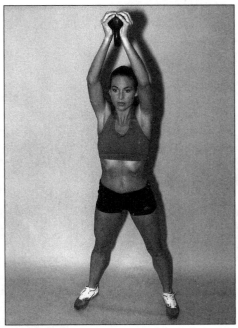

Kettlebell squat and press start/finish position (left). Kettlebell squat and press middle position (right).

Crunch and Punch

Here's a variation on a standard crunch, in which you do a one-armed chest press at the same time. Once again, you get lots of muscle recruitment in one exercise.

1. Begin in a crunch position, with one hand behind your head (for support) and the other holding a kettlebell.

2. Rest the kettlebell by your shoulder.

3. As you perform a crunch, press the weight toward the ceiling.

Coordinate the movement so your shoulder blades return to the mat as the kettlebell is lowered back to your shoulder.

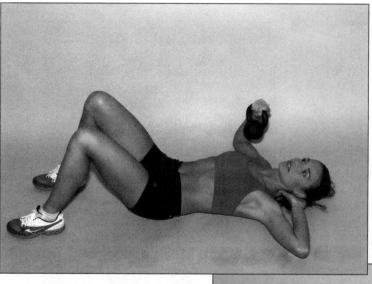

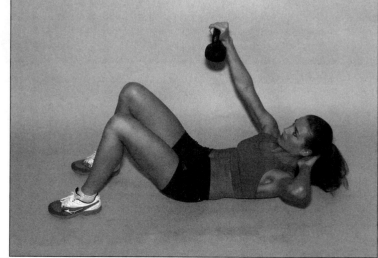

Kettlebell crunch and punch start/finish position (top). Kettlebell crunch and punch middle position (bottom).

Single-Leg Romanian Deadlift

This one sounds old school because it is. Use it to strengthen your lower back and hips. Avoid it if you have a history of lower back problems.

1. Begin in a narrow stance, with a kettlebell in one hand.

2. Keep the foot opposite the kettlebell down, while lifting the other foot.

3. Bending forward at the waist, lower the kettlebell to the ground.

4. Allow the leg and opposite hand to swing behind you as a counterbalance.

5. Return to the standing position.

In addition to working your back and hips, the single-leg Romanian deadlift is great for the muscles in your calves and feet.

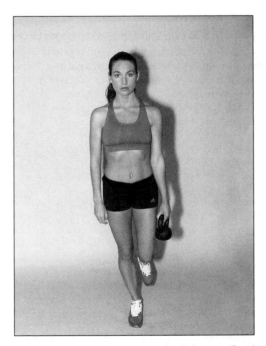 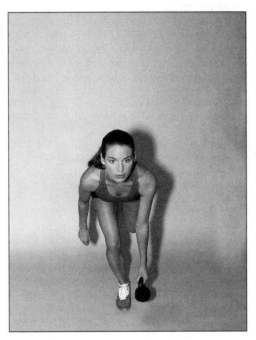

Kettlebell single-leg Romanian deadlift start/finish position (left). Kettlebell single-leg Romanian deadlift middle position (right).

Medicine Balls

Back in the day, there wasn't a lot of variety among medicine balls. Today you'll find them in different sizes and weights, some with handles, some that bounce, and some that don't budge when they hit the ground. This variety allows for an even longer list of exercises you can do with medicine balls. These are a few of our favorites.

Completing a total-body workout using nothing more than a medicine ball may not seem intimidating, but know this: Jonas Sahratian, the strength and conditioning coach at the University of North Carolina, used a 10-exercise routine to whip the Tar Heels into championship-game shape. It's designed to help you build a backboard-firm core, burn fat, and improve your sports performance.

Sahratian calls this workout the Med Ball 400. The 400 represents 400 repetitions—the number players like former Tar Heels star Tyler Hansbrough completed before he headed to the NBA. However, Sahratian suggests you start with 200 reps. (Call it the Med Ball 200.)

SPOT ME

As any fan of the movie *Rocky* recalls, boxers use medicine balls to improve their abs strength by dropping the ball onto the boxer's "bread basket," simulating a punch. Another, less punishing way to improve your core strength is to sit on the floor as if you were doing a crunch and play catch with a partner. This exercise also strengthens arm, chest, and leg muscles.

Medicine Ball Push-ups

There's a reason we keep coming back to push-ups: they're a great exercise. Adding a medicine ball to the exercise introduces some instability to make it more challenging.

1. Assume a standard push-up position, but with a small medicine ball beneath one hand.

2. Perform one repetition.

3. While your arms are straight, roll the medicine ball to the other side and place it under the opposite hand.

4. Repeat.

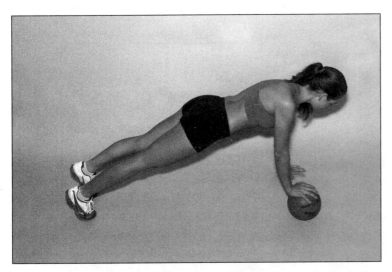

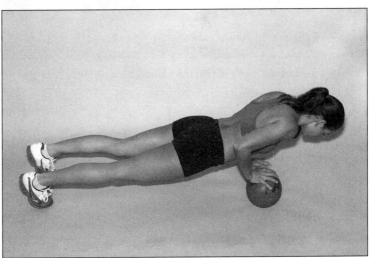

Medicine ball push-ups start/finish position (top). Medicine ball push-ups middle position (bottom).

Split Squat with Rotation

Once again, we go back to one of our favorite exercises, but we throw in a twist. Literally.

1. Assume a split stance—feet parallel, one in front, the other beneath you.

2. Hold a medicine ball in front of you, with your arms parallel to the ground.

3. Bend the front knee, twisting your arms in the direction of the forward leg as you bend it.

4. Return to center and repeat.

5. Switch sides after a full set in one direction.

We favor this exercise because it's effective for your glutes, quads, hamstrings, core, and lots more.

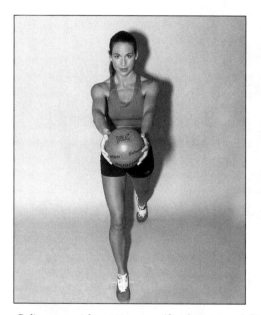 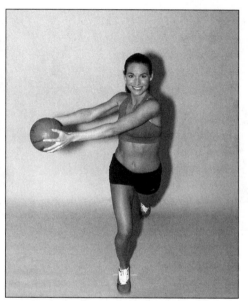

Split squat with rotation start/finish position (left). Split squat with rotation middle position (right).

Russian Twist

This is another exercise with an Eastern European name, and it's also another that's great for your core.

1. Lie on a mat with both knees bent and holding the medicine ball to your chest.

2. Curl into a crunch position.

3. Twist right and then twist left, touching the ball to the floor on each side.

4. Repeat.

To make this exercise more challenging, do it with your feet off the floor.

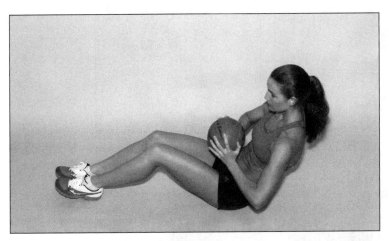

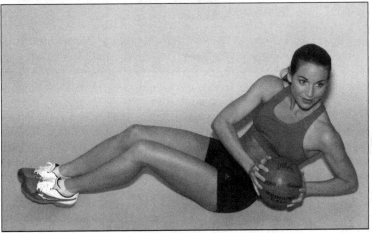

Russian twist start/finish position (top). Russian twist middle position (bottom).

11–1 o'clock

This one may not look as impressive as some of the other medicine ball exercises, but it's an effective way to work on your core.

1. Assume a narrow stance, holding a medicine ball high overhead with your arms straight.

2. Keeping your knees straight and initiating the movement by shifting your hips to the right, move the medicine ball to your left until your arms are in the 11 o'clock position.

3. Return to center.

4. Shift to the opposite side until you reach 1 o'clock.

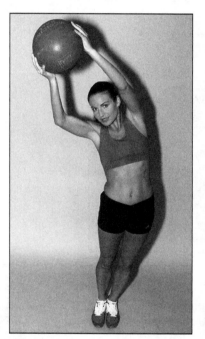 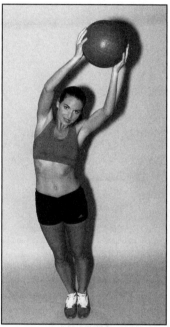

11–1 o'clock start/finish position (left). 11–1 o'clock middle position (right).

Cables

Cables are an effective and versatile strength-training method. They allow you to work in any movement pattern you like and to quickly manipulate the resistance. The amount of weight novice cable users can safely train with is less than they are used to with traditional resistance machines because the machine isn't stabilizing them. Maintaining proper form throughout the exercise is key. But just because you're using less weight doesn't mean you're not getting fitter. Cable training enhances balance, coordination, stability, and kinesthetic awareness.

Core Twist

Here's a great core exercise with cables.

1. Sit on a physioball (remember, we introduced you to those in Chapter 12) with your feet just in front of the ball.

2. Adjust the cable so it's at shoulder height.

3. Hold the cable handle with both hands, arm extended straight in front of you.

4. Twist away from the cable.

5. Return to center.

6. Repeat.

7. Turn 180° degrees and repeat the exercise on the other side.

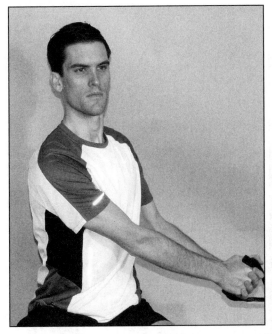

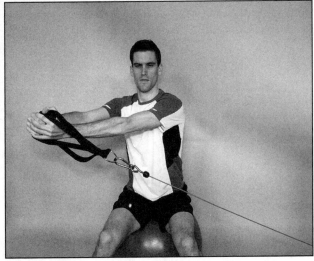

Core twist start/finish position (left). Core twist middle position (right).

Reverse Flye

Most folks spend way too much time hunched over a computer with their shoulders rounded. The reverse flye is a great way to help combat those tight chest muscles, as well as the weakness in the opposing muscles in your back. Don't expect to be able to move much weight in this exercise. That just serves to show you how much it's needed.

1. Begin with the cable handles all the way down.

2. Bend forward from the waist, keeping your knees slightly bent and your feet hip width apart.

3. Grab the left handle with your right hand, and vice versa. (Your arms are crossed.)

4. Keeping a slight bend in your elbows, uncross your arms and raise them to your sides until they're parallel to the ground.

5. Slowly lower and repeat.

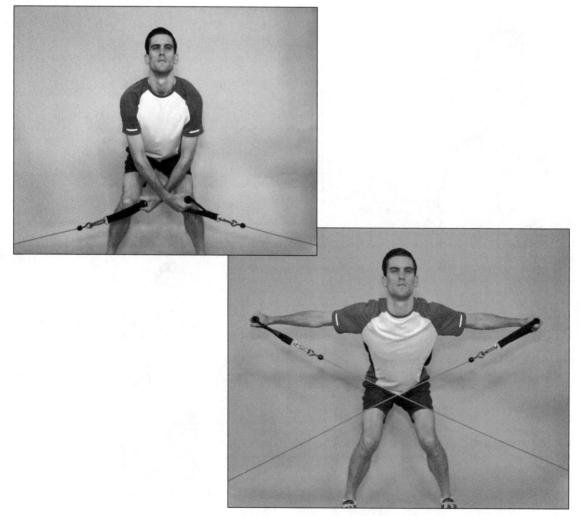

Reverse flye start/finish position (top). Reverse flye middle position (bottom).

The Chop

Good luck doing this with anything other than cables. Thankfully, you don't have to try. And thankfully, this gives your core a great workout.

1. Adjust the cable so it's at the top of your reach.

2. Grab the handle with both hands.

3. Keep your eyes on the handles.

4. Maintaining straight arms, bring the cable down toward the opposite hip in a chopping motion.

5. End the motion with both knees bent and both hands by the hip opposite the column.

6. Repeat.

7. Switch sides.

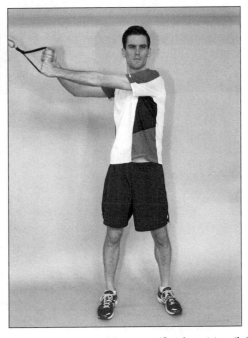 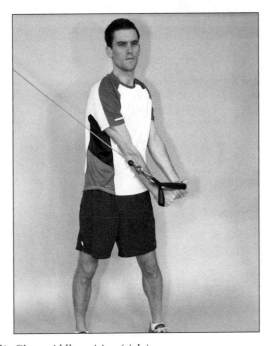

Chop start/finish position (left). Chop middle position (right).

WEIGHT A MINUTE

Using cable equipment is not as easy as just lifting a free weight or pulling out a pin on a machine. A certain amount of learning is involved in figuring out how to properly use them, how to set them up, and how to stand. But once you get the feel of it, the benefits speak for themselves.

The Toss

Here's another exercise that takes full advantage of the versatile nature of cables.

1. Adjust the cable so it's at the bottom of the column.

2. Bend both knees as you reach for the handle with both hands.

3. Keep your eyes on the cable.

4. As you stand, keep your arms straight and bring them across your chest.

5. End the motion standing with both arms extended in the opposite direction of your starting motion.

6. Repeat.

7. Switch sides.

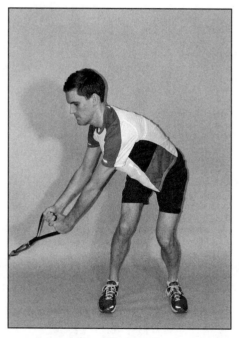 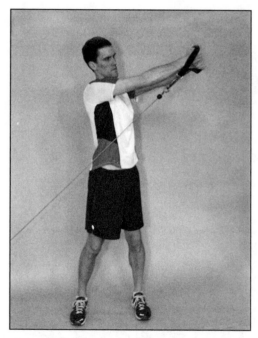

Toss start/finish position (left). Toss middle position (right).

Bands on the Run

In This Chapter

- Maintaining muscles on the road or at home
- Choosing your weapon
- Working out with bands and straps: some great exercises

Free weights and machines are the most conventional and efficient ways to strengthen your muscles, but you can't always get to the gym to use them. If you're on the road, are stuck at work, or for any other reason can't make it to the gym, you don't have to miss your workout altogether. We have two favorite weapons when the gym isn't practical.

In Deidre's physical therapy office, they're known as Therabands. At her gym, they go by Dynabands. Generically, they're called resistance bands. A rose is a rose is a rose, and a resistance band is basically a giant rubber band on steroids. They're color coded according to their level of resistance and can be cut to any length for use in a variety of exercises. Using resistance bands as your sole (or even main) source of strength training won't get you entered in a powerlifting meet anytime soon, nor can you adequately address all the muscles you might want to, but it is a safe, inexpensive, easy way to maintain strength when a gym workout is impractical.

Our other preferred traveling companion—a registered trademark product called TRX Suspension Training—is a simple set of ropes, handles, and foot cradles that allows you to perform one of 3,000 (okay, more like 300) exercises. Favored by pro jocks and fitness trainers hither and yon, it's a comprehensive workout in which body weight is pitted against gravity. Trademarked by Randy Hetrick, a former Navy SEAL, the TRX uses regimens that allow for a variety of movements—from simple one-joint exercises to compound movements (think of a push-up for your chest and back that leads into a crunch for your abs) so that you get an efficient workout.

To weigh the resistance bands pros and cons ...

Pros of Resistance Bands

- Easy to pack.
- Variable resistance. (They come in different grades, and you can pull them looser or tighter.)
- Can be used for a variety of exercises.
- Safe.

Cons of Resistance Bands

- Resistance is not constant throughout the full range of motion. (It's fairly easy at first and gets harder as you pull it tighter.)
- Although effective for some smaller muscle groups, bands are not as useful for larger ones such as your glutes, quads, and hamstrings, where greater resistance is needed.
- They break. Stretch the bands enough times, and they'll wear out.

Pros of TRX

- Very versatile. Almost any exercise you can imagine can be done with TRX.
- Light, easy to pack, and takes just a few seconds to set up.
- Great for doing compound exercises and hitting a lot of muscle groups in one exercise.

Cons of TRX

- A lot of money for such simple materials.
- Hard to do some exercises without assistance.

SPOT ME

The best thing about resistance bands is that they're so portable and easy to use when you're on the road (or even in your office if you can't make it to the gym). We're not saying you'll get in great shape using them exclusively, but their convenience and ease of use makes them a practical way to maintain fitness when a visit to the gym is impossible.

Band Land

Let's start with some band exercises. We don't usually get too fancy with bands. Instead, we mimic conventional free-weight exercises. The trick to using resistance bands is to choose a band with the appropriate level of resistance and to have some tension on the band as you start the exercise. Having some tension means your muscles are firing even at the beginning of the range of motion. If you're in need of a real challenge, you can always fold the band over or use more than one at a time to make the exercise particularly difficult.

FLEX FACTS

Because bands gain tension as they're stretched, their resistance level changes throughout the range of motion. You'll find that exercises are easier at the beginning and harder at the end of the movement. To ensure benefit throughout the range of motion, start the exercise with some tension on the band.

Let's take a look at some of our favorite band exercises.

Band Low Row

The band low row simulates the low cable row, working the muscles of your back and biceps. Here's the drill:

1. Sit on the floor and wrap the band around the balls of your feet.

2. With elbows bent, pull your arms back while squeezing your shoulder blades together.

3. Slowly return to the starting position.

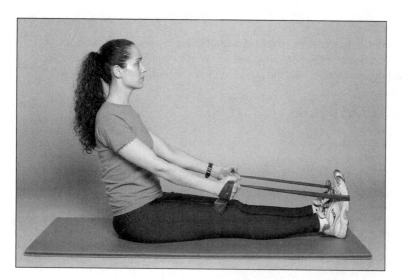

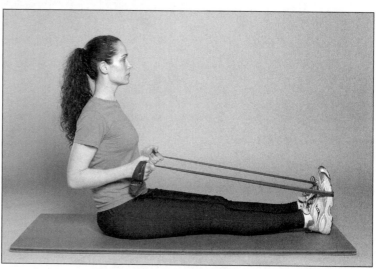

Band low row start/finish position (top). Band low row middle position (bottom).

Band Chest Press

When you can't make it to the gym, this is a great alternate to the bench press. Here's how to properly perform the exercise:

1. Wrap the band around your back.

2. Grip the ends of the band with both hands.

3. Press your arms forward, bringing them together at the end.

4. Slowly return to the starting position.

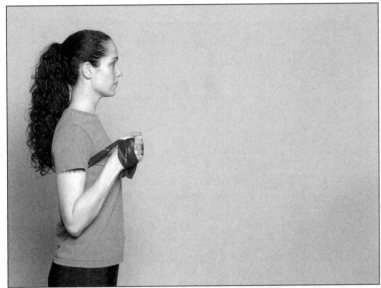

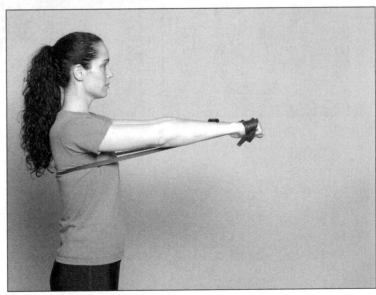

Band chest press start/finish position (top). Band chest press middle position (bottom).

Band Lateral Raise

The band lateral raise is an effective alternative to the free-weight version. Here's what you need to know:

1. Stand with your feet shoulder width apart, and step on the middle of the band.

2. Hold one end of the band in each hand.

3. Maintaining a slight bend in each elbow, slowly raise your arms to the side until they reach shoulder height.

4. Slowly return to the starting position.

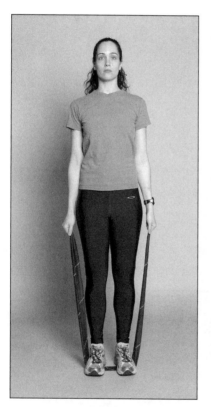 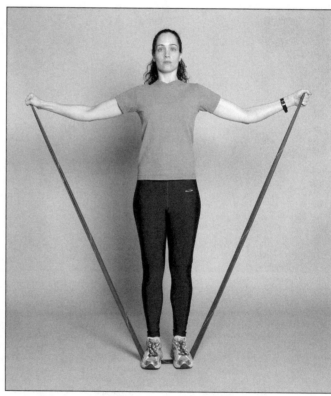

Band lateral raise start/finish position (left). Band lateral raise middle position (bottom).

Band Front Raise

Front raises with a resistance band are quite effective in isolating the anterior part of your deltoid. Here's how to do them properly:

1. Stand with your feet shoulder width apart, and step on the band.

2. Hold one end of the band in one hand.

3. While maintaining proper alignment, slowly raise your arms in front of you until you reach shoulder height.

4. Slowly return to the starting position.

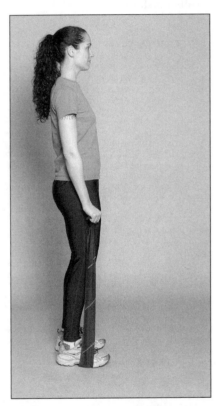 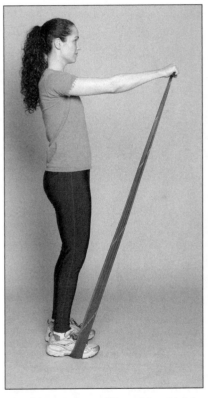

Band front raise start/finish position (left). Band front raise middle position (right).

Band Biceps Curls

You probably won't make it to Muscle Beach with just bands, but using them for biceps curls works in a pinch. Here's how to do them right:

1. Stand with your feet shoulder width apart.

2. Hold each end of the band, and stand on the middle of it.

3. Ensure that there's some tension on the band in the starting position, wrapping it around your hand, if necessary.

4. Slowly curl your hands to your shoulder by bending your elbow.

5. Return to the starting position in a slow, controlled fashion.

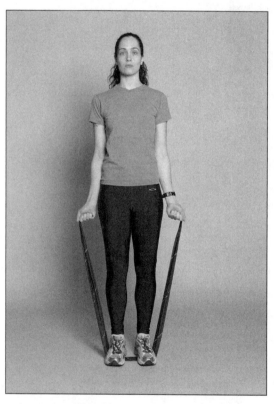 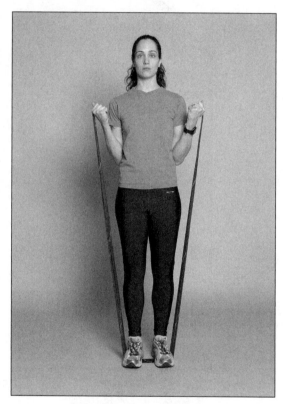

Band biceps curl start/finish position (left). Band biceps curl middle position (right).

Band Triceps Extension

When you've worked your biceps, you always want to train the opposite side of your arm—the triceps. This is what you need to do:

1. Grasp each end of the band with your hands.

2. Hold the nonexercising hand at your side.

3. Bring the exercising hand behind your head, near your opposite shoulder.

4. Keeping your upper arm vertical, raise your exercising hand by straightening your elbow.

5. Slowly return to the starting position.

6. Repeat on the other side.

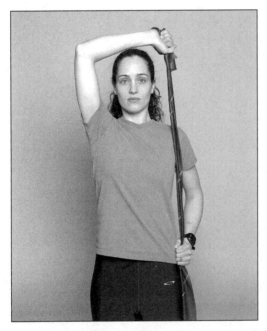 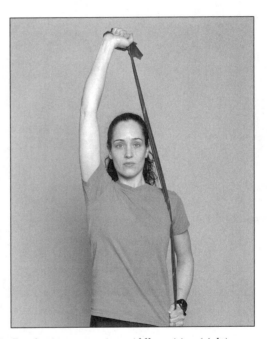

Band triceps extension start/finish position (left). Band triceps extension middle position (right).

SPOT ME

Bands are not our preferred method of resistance for most exercises, but they're perfect for internal and external rotation. Using dumbbells requires you to lie in uncomfortable positions and doesn't allow for tension through the full range of motion; bands, on the other hand, are easy to use in any position.

Band Internal Rotation

Bands are effective for internal and external rotation exercises. These are not flashy or exciting exercises, but they're great for working the muscles of your rotator cuff. Therefore, they're valuable for any athlete who plays racquet or throwing sports. Here are the basics:

1. Securely tie a band around a stable, waist-high object, such as a door knob.

2. Stand with the band at your side.

3. Grasp the end of the band with the hand closest to the secured end.

4. Bend your elbow to 90° and rotate your arm outward.

5. Keeping your elbow pinned against your torso and your shoulders squared, slowly rotate your arm inward.

6. Slowly return to the starting position.

7. Repeat on the other side.

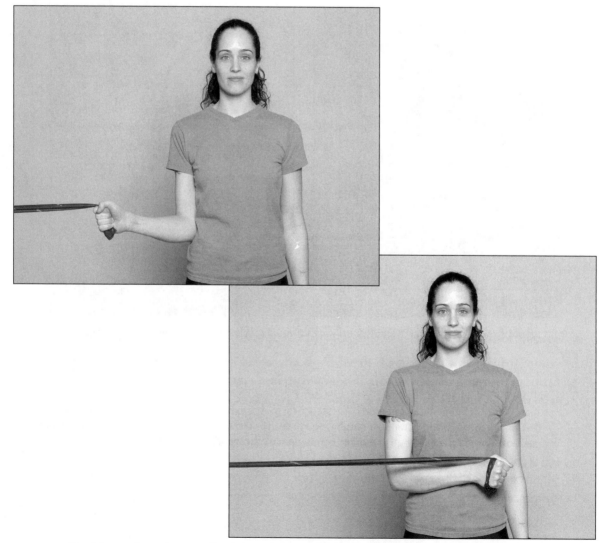

Band internal rotation start/finish position (top). Band internal rotation middle position (bottom).

Band External Rotation

External rotation is the kissin' cousin to internal rotation. It, too, is a great rotator cuff exercise. Here's what to do:

1. Securely tie a band around a stable, waist-high object, such as a door knob.

2. Stand with the band at your side.

3. Grasp the end of the band with the hand farthest from the secured end.

4. Bend your elbow to 90° and rotate your arm inward.

5. Keeping your elbow pinned against your torso and your shoulders squared, slowly rotate your arm outward.

6. Slowly return to the starting position.

7. Repeat on the other side.

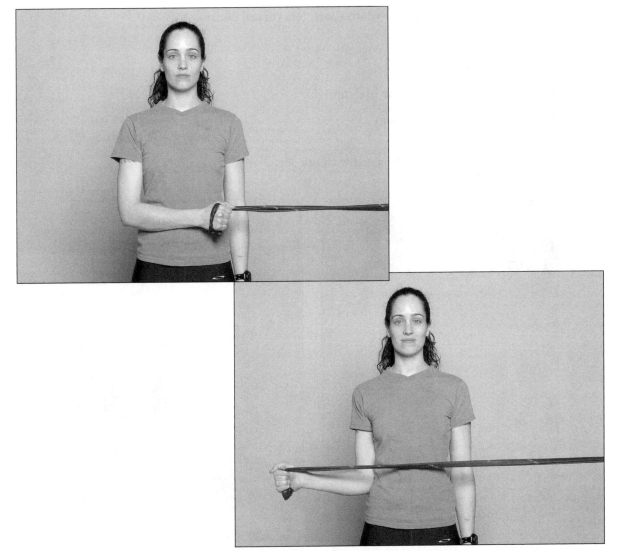

Band external rotation start/finish position (top). Band external rotation middle position (bottom).

Suspend Your Training: TRX

As we mentioned, TRX is versatile, and with a little imagination you can work on just about any muscles you want. Some exercises are like movements you'd do in the gym with free weights or machines, but at other times, you can really "think outside the box." Here are a few ideas.

Squats

They're our favorite free-weight exercise for your legs, and the same goes for the TRX version. You get lots of muscle recruitment in one movement.

1. Face toward the anchor position.

2. Hold the handles.

3. Stand with your legs shoulder width apart, feet turned out slightly.

4. Lean back.

5. Bend knees and hips to 90°.

6. Keep your core tight and your back upright.

7. Return to the starting position.

For an extra challenge, you can try to squat with one leg.

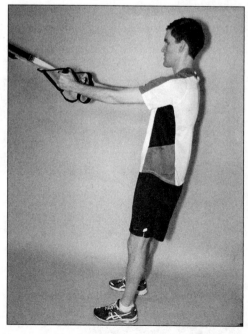 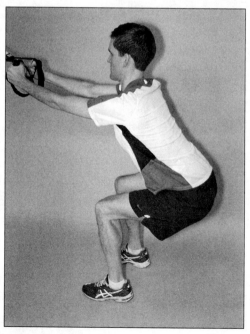

TRX squat start/finish position (left). TRX squat middle position (right).

Chest Press

The TRX chest press is an awesome way to build upper-body strength. It's a simple exercise to set up, but it can be very challenging. Change your body angle to manipulate the resistance.

1. Adjust the handles so they come down to around your knees.

2. Grab the handles.

3. Face away from the anchor position.

4. Tighten your core muscles.

5. Gently lower yourself toward your hands while keeping the spine aligned and not sagging.

6. When your chest is down by your hands, exhale and push back up as if you're doing a bench press.

This is more challenging than a standard bench press because you need to use your core muscles to stabilize yourself and avoid losing control. A more upright starting position makes the exercise easier; keeping your feet back and leaning in increases the challenge.

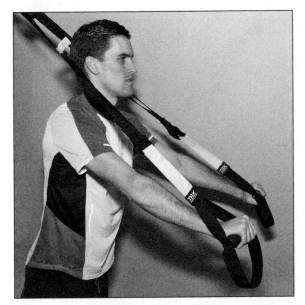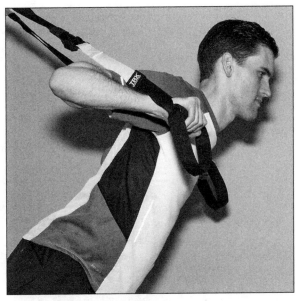

TRX chest press start/finish position (left). TRX chest press middle position (right).

Row

Here's another exercise that's similar to a free weight or machine movement, but it's a real challenge because you need to stabilize yourself by contracting your core muscles.

1. Face the anchor position.

2. Stand with your feet shoulder-width apart.

3. Grab both handles.

4. Stabilize your torso by contracting your core muscles.

5. Gently lean back until your elbows are straight.

6. Exhale and pull your body toward your hands by bending your elbows, squeezing your shoulder blades together at the top.

7. Return to the starting position.

Again, you can vary the resistance by changing your foot placement. The farther forward your feet are, the harder the exercise is.

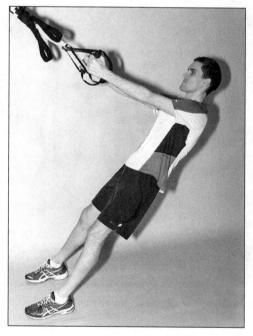 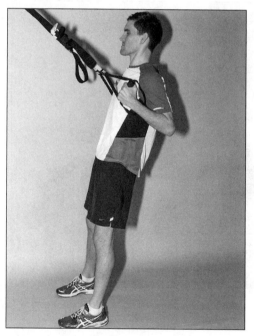

TRX row start/finish position (left). TRX row middle position (right).

Suspended Pushup

Here's a challenging variation on an old favorite.

1. Start with your feet in the foot cradles directly under the anchor position.

2. To maintain stability in the cradles, push down with your feet by pointing your toes.

3. Lie flat, face down, with your hands under your shoulders facing forward.

4. Engage your core muscles.

5. Exhale and slowly press your body off the floor until your elbows are straight.

6. Slowly return to starting position, being sure to keep your spine straight and your core muscles contracted.

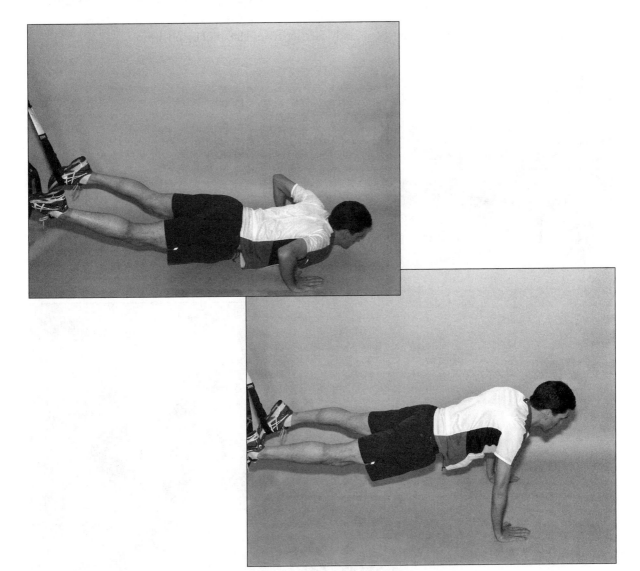

TRX suspended pushup start/finish position (top). TRX suspended pushup middle position (bottom).

Knee Tucks

TRX is especially effective for core exercises. This is one of the best.

1. Start with your feet in the foot cradles, directly under the anchor position.

2. To maintain stability in the cradles, push down with the tops of your feet and point your toes.

3. Begin in a plank position with your body suspended and your hands on the floor, shoulder width apart.

4. Keeping your feet together, slowly pull your knees toward your chest, bending your knees as they tuck under your hips.

5. Allow your hips to rise as your spine rounds.

6. Slowly lower your body to plank position. Be sure to maintain a rigid core and keep your lower back from sagging.

You can vary the resistance by moving your body farther from the anchor position.

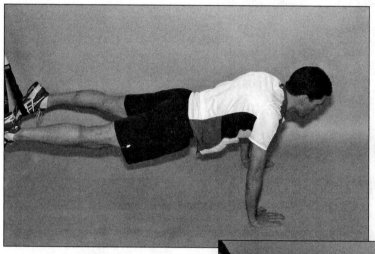

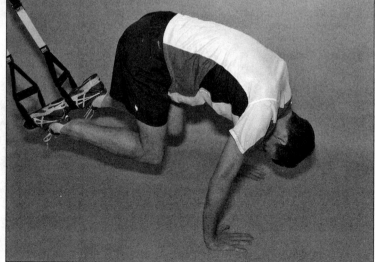

TRX knee tucks start/finish position (top). TRX knee tucks middle position (bottom).

abdominals (abs)   Muscles of the midsection.

abduction   Sideways movement away from the body.

abductors   Muscles that move your leg away from your body.

adduction   Sideways movement in the direction toward the body.

adductors   Muscles that draw your leg in toward your body from an outward position.

aerobic   Exercise that requires a significant and sustained supply of oxygen. Literally means "in the presence of oxygen."

amino acids   The structural material or "building blocks" of protein.

anaerobic   Exercise that can take place in the absence of oxygen.

anterior   The front of the body.

atrophy   The loss of size of a muscle. The opposite of hypertrophy.

barbell   A straight free weight on which plates can be added for increased resistance.

bench press   A powerlifting exercise that involves lying on your back and pushing a weight from your chest.

biceps   The muscle in the front of the upper arm, responsible for bending (flexing) the elbow.

cables   Adjustable pulley system.

cardiovascular exercise   Any activity that improves your cardiovascular system. Your body's cardiovascular system includes your heart, lungs, and circulatory system.

carpal tunnel syndrome   A condition that is often caused by repetitive activities done with improper body mechanics, such as typing with your wrists in an extended position, or repetitive squeezing activities. The median nerve swells and is unable to pass comfortably through the small bones in your wrist (carpals). Symptoms of carpal tunnel syndrome are numbness, tingling, and a sharp, shooting pain into the hand.

collar   A safety device that helps secure plates on a barbell.

compound movement   An exercise, such as the bench press, squat, or lat pull-down, that involves the movement of more than one joint at a time.

concentric contraction   The shortening of a muscle as it exerts force.

contract   To draw together or shorten. When contracted, a muscle shortens and produces movement.

contracture   A condition in which a joint (shoulder, elbow, wrist, finger, hip, knee, or ankle) is unable to be fully straightened or fully bent.

core   Several muscle groups that together enhance strength, stability, and support for posture.

deadlift   A powerlifting maneuver in which the weighted bar is on the floor, and the lifter bends the knees and hips to reach the bar and then lifts it to midthigh.

delayed onset muscle soreness (DOMS)   The temporary, post-workout pain you feel in your muscles, usually within 24 hours of your workout. It peaks after 48 hours.

deltoid   Major muscle of the shoulder. Divided into medial, posterior, and anterior sections.

diaphragm   A muscle used in respiration.

dumbbell   A handheld free weight.

eccentric contraction   A lengthening of the muscle as it exerts force but is overcome by the resistance.

erector spinae   Muscles of the back that run along the spine.

ergogenic aid   Any product that improves athletic or physical performance.

extend   To increase the angle between body parts, as in straightening the elbow or knee.

fast-twitch muscle fiber   A powerful, easily fatigued muscle fiber.

female athletic triad   A phenomenon common among competitive female athletes that consists of eating disorders, amenorrhea (absence of the menstrual flow), and osteoporosis.

flex   To decrease the angle between body parts, as in bending the elbow or knee. (Commonly, but incorrectly, used to refer to contracting a muscle.)

free weight   A handheld weight, such as a barbell or dumbbell.

gastrocnemius   A muscle in the back of the lower leg, responsible for raising the heel over the toe, especially when the knee is straight.

gluteus (glutes)   The gluteus maximus (the gluteus medius and gluteus minimus are much smaller and weaker), responsible for extension of the hip.

hamstrings   Muscles in the back of the upper leg, responsible for bending the knee and extending the hip. Made up of the biceps femoris, semitendinosus, and semimembranosus muscles.

hyperextend   To extend a joint beyond straight.

hyperplasia   An increase in the amount of muscle fibers in some animals. Does not appear to occur in humans.

hypertrophy   The growth of a muscle and the individual fibers that make it up. This growth usually occurs as a result of an external stimulus such as weightlifting.

impingement   The pinching or squeezing of the internal structures of the shoulder (tendons of the rotator cuff, bursa, ligaments, and nerves). This pinching causes pain on elevation of the arm.

isolation exercise   A lift that uses only one joint, and therefore focuses on one muscle.

isometric contraction   A muscle action that results in no movement because the muscle force and the resistance are equal.

kettlebell   Cast-iron weight that looks like a cannonball with a handle.

lactic acid   A byproduct of anaerobic work that causes fatigue and a burning sensation.

latissimus dorsi (lats)   The large, fan-shaped muscles of the middle and upper back.

ligaments   The connective tissue between bones.

lordosis   The natural inward curve of the lumbar or lower spine.

medicine ball   A large, heavy, solid ball thrown and caught for exercise.

muscle pull   See *muscle strain*.

muscle strain   A trauma to the muscle or tendon caused by excessive contraction or stretching.

overtraining   A phenomenon that occurs when you exercise excessively without allowing sufficient recovery between workouts.

palpitations   An abnormally rapid throbbing or fluttering of the heart.

pectorals (pecs)   The large muscles in the chest.

phlebitis   An inflammation of a vein.

plates   Weighted discs added to a bar to increase its weight. Plates most often come in denominations of 2½, 5, 10, 25, 35, and 45 pounds.

posing   A facet of bodybuilding in which the competitor demonstrates his or her physical assets by assuming various positions that show off muscularity and proportion.

posterior   The rear of the body.

pronation   Turning the hand so the palm faces downward. Opposite of supination.

quadriceps   Muscles of the front of the upper leg, responsible for straightening the knee. Made up of the rectus femoris, vastus lateralis, vastus intermedius, and vastus medialis muscles.

range of motion (ROM)   The movement from the beginning to the finishing point of an exercise. Moving a joint from complete extension to complete flexion is considered a full range of motion.

recovery   The rest period between two sets or workouts.

repetition (rep)   The execution of an exercise one time. Consecutive repetitions are grouped into a set.

Romanian deadlift   A form of deadlift in which the body is bent at the hips and the knees are not bent.

rotator cuff   Group of muscles (supraspinatus, infraspinatus, teres minor, and subscapularis) located under the deltoid.

set   A series of repetitions performed consecutively.

slow-twitch muscle fiber   A muscle fiber that has great endurance but relatively low power.

soleus   A muscle in the back of the lower leg, responsible for raising the heel over the toe, especially when the knee is bent.

spotter   Someone who stands by to help the lifter if and when he or she can't finish a repetition. The spotter is responsible for the lifter's safety.

sprain   Damage due to overstretching of ligaments.

squat   A powerlifting maneuver that involves performing a deep knee bend with a barbell across your back.

sticking point   A particular position during your range of motion in which you have difficulty completing the repetition without assistance.

supination   Turning the hand so the palm faces upward. Opposite of pronation.

T cells   The cells responsible for enhancing antibody production and for killing foreign cells in the body.

tendinitis   A condition characterized by inflammation of a tendon.

tendon   Connective tissue that attaches muscle to bone.

trapezius (traps)   The muscle that covers the rear of the neck and shoulders.

triceps   The muscle in the back of the upper arm, responsible for straightening (extending) the elbow.

TRX   A form of exercise training that involves portable suspension cables and bodyweight.

Valsalva maneuver   Holding the breath while lifting. May lead to excessive increase in blood pressure and decrease in blood returning to the heart.

VO₂ max   A measure of an individual's capacity for aerobic work. It is generally considered one of the most important factors in predicting an athlete's ability to perform in activities of more than 3 to 5 minutes.

weight belt   A thick, wide, dense leather belt used for added support for the lower back when lifting.

working in   The practice of alternating sets on a particular bench or machine with another person.

Resources

Aerobics and Fitness Association of America (AFAA)
15250 Ventura Boulevard, Suite 200
Sherman Oaks, CA 91403
877-YOURBODY (877-968-7263)
www.afaa.com

American College of Sports Medicine (ACSM)
401 West Michigan Street
Indianapolis, IN 46202-3233
317-637-9200
www.acsm.org

American Council on Exercise (ACE)
4851 Paramount Drive
San Diego, CA 92123
858-279-8227 or 800-825-3636
www.acefitness.org

Athletic Business
4130 Lien Road
Madison, WI 53704
608-249-0186
www.athleticbusiness.com

Concept II
105 Industrial Park Drive
Morrisville, VT 05661-9727
800-245-5676
www.concept2.com

Cyberpump
www.cyberpump.com

Cybex International, Inc.
10 Trotter Drive
Medway, MA 02053
508-533-4300
cybex.com

Gatorade Sports Science Institute
617 W. Main Street
Barrington, IL 60010
800-616-GSSI (800-616-4774)
www.gssiweb.com

Healthclubs.com
www.healthclubs.com

Healthfinder
www.healthfinder.gov

LifeFitness
5100 North River Road
Schiller Park, Il 60176
800-527-6063
www.lifefitness.com

Nancy Clark Sports Nutrition
www.nancyclarkrd.com

National Strength and Conditioning Association (NSCA)
1885 Bob Johnson Drive
Colorado Springs, CO 80906
800-815-6826
www.nsca-cc.org

National Strength Professionals Association (NSPA)
P.O. Box 967
Mount Airy, MD 21771
410-635-2235
www.nspainc.com

Natural Strength
www.naturalstrength.com

Nautilus, Inc.
Global Headquarters
16400 SE Nautilus Drive
Vancouver, WA 98683
800-628-8458
www.nautilusinc.com

Polar
1111 Marcus Avenue, Suite M15
Lake Success, NY 11042-1034
800-227-1314
www.polarusa.com

PowerBlock
PowerBlock, Inc.
1071 32nd Avenue NW
Owatonna, MN 55060
507-451-5152
www.powerblock.com

Power Systems, Inc.
5700 Casey Drive
Knoxville, TN 37909
800-321-6975
www.power-systems.com

Precor
20031 142nd Avenue NE
P.O. Box 7202
Woodinville, WA 98072-4002
800-786-8404
www.precor.com

StairMaster Sports
12421 Willows Road NE, Suite 100
Kirkland, WA 98034
888-678-2476
www.stairmaster.com

Star Trac
14410 Myford Road
Irvine, CA 92606
800-745-3815
www.startrac.com

Total Gym
7755 Arjons Drive
San Diego, CA 92126
800-541-4900
www.totalgym.com

TRX
755 Sansome Street, 6th Floor
San Francisco, CA 94111
888-878-5348
www.trxtraining.com

U.S. Food and Drug Administration (FDA)
10903 New Hampshire Avenue
Silver Spring, MD 20993
888-INFO-FDA (888-463-6332)
www.fda.gov

VersaClimber Heart Rate, Inc.
1411 E. Wilshire Avenue
Santa Ana, CA 92705
800-237-2271
www.versaclimber.com

Women's Sports Foundation
Eisenhower Park
1899 Hempstead Turnpike, Suite 400
East Meadow, NY 11554
800-227-3988
www.womenssportsfoundation.org

Index

D

CHECK OUT THESE BEST-SELLERS

More than 450 titles available at booksellers and online retailers everywhere!

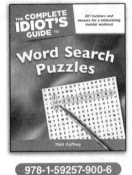

THE COMPLETE **IDIOT'S GUIDE** TO

Rights and wrongs of sentence structure, word usage, spelling, and much more

Grammar & Style
SECOND EDITION

Laurie E. Rozakis, Ph.D.

978-1-59257-115-4

THE COMPLETE **IDIOT'S GUIDE** TO

301 twisters and teasers for a stimulating mental workout

Word Search Puzzles

Matt Gaffney

978-1-59257-900-6

THE COMPLETE **IDIOT'S GUIDE** TO

Rev up your metabolism and lose weight—for good

Glycemic Index Weight Loss
SECOND EDITION

Lucy Beale and Joan Clark-Warner, M.S., R.D., C.D.E.

978-1-59257-855-9

THE COMPLETE **IDIOT'S GUIDE** TO

A revealing comparison of the faiths that shape the lives of millions

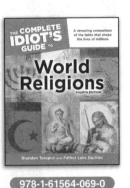

World Religions
FOURTH EDITION

Brandon Toropov and Father Luke Buckles

978-1-61564-069-0

THE COMPLETE **IDIOT'S GUIDE** TO

Give your resume a professional makeover—and stand out from the pack

The Perfect Resume
FIFTH EDITION

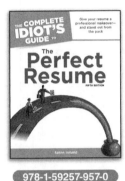

Susan Ireland

978-1-59257-957-0

THE COMPLETE **IDIOT'S GUIDE** TO

A lively, comprehensive guide to the dramatic history of our great nation

American History
FIFTH EDITION

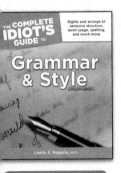

Alan Axelrod, Ph.D.

978-1-59257-869-6

THE COMPLETE **IDIOT'S GUIDE** TO

Calculus
SECOND EDITION

Sail through class with foolproof explanations and dozens of practice problems

W. Michael Kelley

978-1-59257-471-1

THE COMPLETE **IDIOT'S GUIDE** TO

Easy, effective, and enjoyable methods for you and your dog

Positive Dog Training
THIRD EDITION

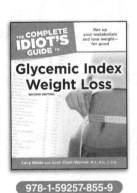

Pamela Dennison

978-1-61564-066-9

THE COMPLETE **IDIOT'S GUIDE** TO

Money-management tips and investment strategies to put your money in your pocket

Personal Finance in Your 20s & 30s
FOURTH EDITION

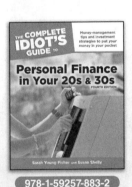

Sarah Young Fisher and Susan Shelly

978-1-59257-883-2

THE COMPLETE **IDIOT'S GUIDE** TO

Tips and tricks to getting your house in order—one room at a time

Organizing Your Life
FIFTH EDITION

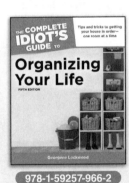

Georgene Lockwood

978-1-59257-966-2

🔵 **CD INCLUDED!**

THE COMPLETE **IDIOT'S GUIDE** TO

Audio exercises let you listen, learn, and practice.

Learning Spanish
FIFTH EDITION

Step-by-step lessons help you speak Spanish like a native

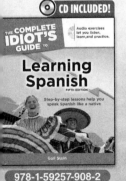

Gail Stein

978-1-59257-908-2

THE COMPLETE **IDIOT'S GUIDE** TO

Refine your taste for the finest in *vino*

Wine Basics
SECOND EDITION

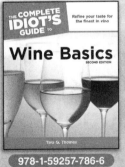

Tara Q. Thomas

978-1-59257-786-6

THE COMPLETE **IDIOT'S GUIDE** TO

Make friends with the social network

Facebook®
SECOND EDITION

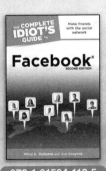

Mikal E. Belicove and Joe Kraynak

978-1-61564-118-5

🔵 **CD INCLUDED!**

THE COMPLETE **IDIOT'S GUIDE** TO

Audio CD
The Complete Idiot's Guide® Ear Training Course

Music Theory
SECOND EDITION

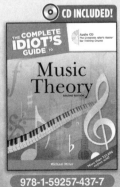

Michael Miller

978-1-59257-437-7

THE COMPLETE **IDIOT'S GUIDE** TO

"Honest, easy-forward advice that will guide you easily through your Walt Disney World vacation."

Walt Disney World
2012 EDITION

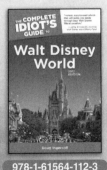

Doug Ingersoll

978-1-61564-112-3

△ ALPHA

idiotsguides.com

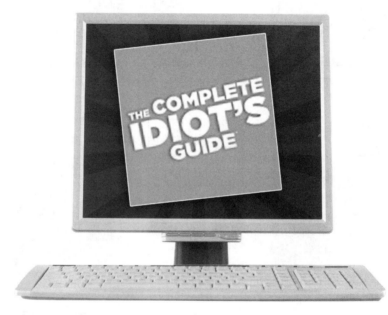